LabCorp

LabCorp

THE DNA OF A CORPORATION

DON BOLDEN

WITH DR. JIM POWELL

CHAPEL HILL

FULL-SERVICE BOOK-MAKERS

ESTD. 1999

PRESS

FRONT COVER PHOTO

Corporate headquarters, Mac Mahon Building in Burlington NC.

BACK COVER PHOTO

Laboratory operations in York Court facilities in Burlington NC.

PUBLISHED BY

The Chapel Hill Press, Inc., Chapel Hill, NC

Hardcover ISBN 978-1-59715-161-0

Paperback ISBN 978-1-59715-150-4

Library of Congress Catalog Number 2017936603

First Printing

Printed in the United States of America

CONTENTS

ACKNOWLEDGMENTS

The material in this book came from the personal files of Dr. James B. Powell, from LabCorp publications, from company news releases, from the pages of the Burlington Times-News and from personal interviews with many of those who have been a part of the LabCorp story dating back to 1969. Photographs also came from Dr. Powell's files as well as from LabCorp. Special appreciation goes to Jay Massengill, a photographer on the LabCorp staff for the past 29 years, now working in the Burlington headquarters. He made many of the photos in the book, and he made the color photographs on the front and back covers of the book.

INTRODUCTION

In the pages that follow is the story of a company that personifies the ideal of American entrepreneurship. LabCorp (Laboratory Corporation of America) is a world leading life sciences company.

It had its beginning in three rooms of the basement of an abandoned hospital in a small North Carolina town, and as the company approaches its fiftieth anniversary, it employs over fifty thousand people and revenues for 2016 were over $9 billion.

Here you will meet many of the people who helped make all this happen. You will read of their willingness to do whatever had to be done to make their company grow. You will read of successes as well as some significant challenges.

You will see the impact of visionary leadership; the company has had only three CEOs in its nearly fifty-year history. You will see the value placed on creating leadership from within, and you will see how this company has helped doctors all across the nation better serve their patients, whose lives are made better in the process.

Today, LabCorp is still on the move, growing its footprint not only in the United States but in foreign countries as well, preparing itself to be a major factor in world health care as time goes on, assuring better health and better lives for generations to come.

Just as this company could not have succeeded without Dr. Jim Powell, this book could not have been done without him either. It was his idea, and he has provided tremendous resources toward its production. Many others have helped eagerly to make this book possible. My thanks to each one.

I appreciate Jim Powell giving me the opportunity to write this book. I like to tell a good story, and this is one of the best that has come my way.

Don Bolden

CHAPTER ONE

The Seeds of Entrepreneurship

IN 1987 A YOUNG BURLINGTON, NORTH CAROLINA, man was in prison working desperately to prove his innocence of crimes he said he did not commit.

Ronald Cotton's prospects for the future could not have been worse at that time. Two years earlier, in July 1985, Cotton had been convicted of rape and burglary. He was sentenced to life in prison plus fifty-four years. An appeal brought him a new trial in 1987, but again the jury found him guilty not only in the original case but also in a second one, which had happened that same night in 1984. Cotton was sentenced again to life in prison, plus fifty-four years on both charges.

Prosecutors said that a couple of things tied him to the case—a flashlight found at his home and traces of rubber found at the scene that were consistent with rubber from Cotton's shoes. The issue that cemented the case, however, was Cotton's identification by one of the victims. That victim, Jennifer Thompson, picked Cotton out of a photo lineup, and then she made the same identification in a live lineup. She was positive—absolutely positive—Cotton was the man who had broken into her apartment and raped her. The victim later said she made every effort to study the attacker so that she could identify him for police should she survive the attack.

Cotton's attorneys made several efforts at appeal, but nothing was found that could give the young man any hope.

Then, in 1995, Burlington police gave all evidence in the case to the defense. Alamance County attorney Tom Lambeth and Richard Rosen, University of North

Carolina law professor emeritus, were handling the case by then, and they believed that a new test might be of value to Cotton. DNA testing was being done in some cases, but up until that time, the new testing had not reached a level that gave it a major role in crime investigations. In fact, about the time that Cotton was charged in 1985, law enforcement was just beginning to use DNA in the apprehension of criminals. As time passed, those in law enforcement began to realize they had a valuable new tool to help them solve even the most difficult cases. But while DNA could help bring conviction in the toughest cases, those in the justice system also learned that DNA could be used to prove the innocence of individuals who might have been wrongly charged.

Cotton learned about DNA himself while in prison. He had a radio in his cell and heard about it in the O. J. Simpson trial. He heard that DNA was 99 percent reliable. That gave him hope.

With that same hope, Lambeth and Rosen went to the prison camp in Harnett County, North Carolina, where Cotton was located at the time. They talked to him about DNA and told him there might be a chance it could prove his innocence. They told him, however, it could also prove him guilty.

Cotton said, "Test it!"

Rob Johnson was district attorney in Alamance County at the time, and when approached about agreeing to such a test, he said yes because he had no interest in keeping an innocent man in prison. The investigating detective in the case, Mike Gaulding, was also very cooperative.

Alamance County Superior Court Judge Jack Spencer signed the order for the test, and Ronald Cotton had a new chance at freedom.

The plan was to have the test done by the lab of the State Bureau of Investigation, with LabCorp, a Burlington-based medical testing laboratory, looking over the state's shoulder. But after seeing LabCorp's operation and its much newer equipment, SBI decided that LabCorp would do the test. Dr. Marcia Eisenberg of LabCorp was given the lead in the laboratory testing of the evidence.

The test revealed absolutely no link between the sample and Ronald Cotton. When that sample was sent to the State Bureau of Investigation labs, a match was found with a convict already in prison—an individual who had told another inmate that he had committed the Burlington crimes.

In June 1995 Ronald Cotton was returned to the Alamance County courtroom where he had been convicted, and Superior Court Judge J. B. Allen Jr. told Cotton that he was a free man. All charges were dropped, and a month later the governor of North Carolina pardoned the young man.

It was ironic that Cotton was in the same prison at one time with the man who actually did the crime, and Cotton said that at one time he shaped a weapon and intended to kill that man. However, he said, his father visited him, learned of his plan, and told his son, "You say you are innocent, but if you kill this man you will be guilty." So Cotton threw the weapon away.

Cotton's story drew national attention not only because of his gaining his freedom but because of the friendship that developed between him and the young woman whose identification had sent him to prison.

When they met for the first time after Cotton's release at a church in Elon, North Carolina, just outside Burlington, Thompson broke into tears and asked if he could somehow find it in his heart to forgive her, but he replied through his own tears that he had forgiven her a long time ago. Since then they have traveled the country talking about wrongful convictions and wrongful identifications and how they might be prevented in other cases in the future. The two have appeared on national television's top news and talk shows, including *60 Minutes* and *The Larry King Show,* and they collaborated in publishing *Picking Cotton: Our Memoir of Injustice and Redemption.* Thompson has created Healing Justice, an organization that speaks to the cases like the one in which she and Cotton were involved. She has worked with legislative bodies in several states to advance compensation laws for the wrongly convicted. Today Thompson and Cotton remain best of friends.

The case continues to make news. In 2016 the North Carolina Press Association named Thompson its 2016 North Carolinian of the Year. Also in that same year, at the invitation of the Burlington School, the two came back to Burlington and told their story in the city where that story had its beginning.

Ironically, when Cotton sought a job after his release and pardon, he found one with LabCorp, the company that had proved his innocence. He married, had a child, made a home for his family, and moved on with his life.

The Cotton DNA case represents just one of millions of medical tests that LabCorp has processed across the nation over its almost half a century of operations from its home base in the Piedmont of North Carolina. While the Cotton case gave a man back his life, other tests have allowed and continue to allow patients all across the nation to receive proper medical treatment in a prompt and efficient manner

In the years that followed there would be many more cases in which prisoners were freed due to DNA testing—people who had been wrongly convicted, often based on an erroneous identification, as was Ronald Cotton. A number of major murder cases would be solved through DNA tests as well. One in particular was the Green River serial murders on the West Coast, in which an individual was arrested and charged in more than forty murders. For a long time it went unsolved, but when DNA testing was introduced, the case came to a successful end, like a number of others.

The Cotton case did more than draw attention to DNA testing. It brought positive national attention to the company that did the testing.

LabCorp had been operating quietly with its headquarters in Burlington, North Carolina, for a number of years, performing a wide variety of medical tests for an equally wide variety of clients, including doctors, their patients, hospitals, the military, pharmaceutical companies, and law enforcement agencies, among others.

LabCorp resulted from the merger of various small companies over the years. Operating as LabCorp, the company continued growing until it became the largest laboratory testing company in the world. As of 2016 the company is performing tests on some 447,000 specimens daily for an estimated 220,000 clients. The company employs 50,000 people around the world. Among those employees are individuals with expertise in genomics, clinical and anatomic pathology, and many other areas of medicine and science.

Every day LabCorp personnel deal with testing for allergies, cardiology, oncology, dermatology, pain management, obstetrics/gynecology, and others, and those tests are carried out quickly and efficiently with results returned to the clients in a matter of hours to better deal with the problems at hand. For a patient to give blood samples and then get a call from his or her medical provider the next day, with the results and the doctor's plan for any necessary treatment, is today a matter of routine. Those tests are a commonplace tool in today's medical practice.

For many people those tests are literally matters of life or death, and speed in getting test results is essential to their well-being. But speed in testing was not always so good.

Looking for a Better Way

In one branch of the family tree of the LabCorp organization, there appears the story of a young medical student in the 1960s who became frustrated with the medical testing process and decided there had to be a better way.

James B. Powell, a Burlington, North Carolina, native, was a medical student at Duke University, and as part of his work he had to draw blood from patients for thyroid tests. The samples had to be placed in acid-washed glassware and then taken to the basement of the medical school to be prepared for mailing to a laboratory for testing. Samples taken by Powell and the other students were sent to Bioscience Laboratories in Van Nuys, California. That process took up to two weeks, and more often than not, by the time results were returned, the patient had begun treatment without the results or had been released from the hospital.

One day in 1963, as Powell wrestled with his frustration on this lack of speed in processing lab samples, an idea flashed in his mind. At that moment, the story that would lead to the formation of the largest testing laboratory in the world had its beginning.

Why can't there be a laboratory on the East Coast? he asked himself. And why can't that laboratory be in North Carolina?

Soon thereafter the journey that resulted in the formation of an East Coast laboratory began when Powell and his two brothers, Ed and Jim's twin brother, John, and friend Ernie Knesel opened Biomedical Laboratories in the Powells' hometown of Burlington, North Carolina.

Operations began in a building that formerly served as Alamance General Hospital. That facility came available when Alamance Memorial Hospital opened in 1961 and Alamance General was closed. Those vacated facilities were eventually purchased by Dr. Thomas E. Powell Jr., father of Ed, Jim, and John. The elder Dr. Powell had been a professor at Elon College and the founder of Carolina Biological Supply Co. near the college. His success in launching Carolina Biological Supply Co. provided incentive to his sons to move forward with their own ideas.

Dr. Powell had been teaching geology and biology at Elon College (now Elon University) when he found it difficult to find the necessary specimens and materials needed in his teaching. He envisioned a company that would supply products needed to teach biology. His idea became reality in 1927 when he formed his company just east of the college campus while continuing his teaching duties. As time passed, his company grew into the largest supplier of biological teaching products in the nation.

When his three sons came along, he envisioned each of them earning their PhDs in the biological sciences and then joining him in the operations of Carolina Biological Supply Co. He had a highly successful business, and like many successful fathers, he saw his sons stepping in to carry on the company he had prepared for them. Based on his own background, Dr. Powell instilled in his sons an appreciation for hard work, education, and entrepreneurship.

Dr. Powell Knew Hard Work

Dr. Thomas E. Powell Jr. was born on a farm in Warren County, North Carolina, on July 6, 1899, and he grew up in a world of hard farm work, long hours in the fields, and few conveniences. It was a life he did not like, and he knew early on that he wanted something better.

But his life was shaped there as the only son of Thomas E. Powell Sr. and Clara Bobbitt Powell. His grandfathers both served in the Civil War. John Burwell Powell was in the 43rd North Carolina Regiment, serving in the entire war and being part of the surrender at Appomattox. Miles Bobbitt served in the 1st North Carolina Calvary Regiment. He also served in the entire war and was at Appomattox as well.

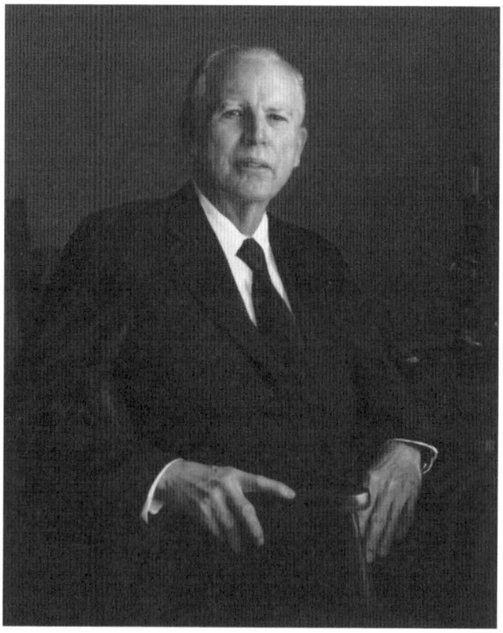

Dr. Thomas E. Powell Jr.

While the young Powell worked hard on that farm in the community of Warren Plains, he grew determined that he would leave those fields and gain an education that would give him a better life. His oldest sister, Mary Powell Brantley, received her college degree at Women's College in Greensboro, now the University of North Carolina at Greensboro. Mary became a teacher and also mentored her brother and sisters. Each of the sisters earned college and master's degrees and followed Mary in teaching.

Mary also encouraged her brother in his studies and in fact helped him financially when he went to Elon. Without her help, he might not have been able to go. Her support proved a good investment as young Tom excelled in his college work. While a student at Macon High School in Warren County, Thomas also had a teacher who urged him to go to Elon College and further his education. So it was that when he was fifteen years old, he took the train to Elon College and began his college education. After he left that day for Elon College, he never returned to Warren County for any length of time.

While he was a student at Elon, the United States entered the "great war" that we later came to know as World War I. It had been raging across Europe for several years. Elon College established a unit of students who wanted to volunteer for officer training courses. Those courses were sponsored at Elon College by the federal government to help fill the need for army officers in the war. The United States had entered the war late, and there was an urgent need for officers, so the young men completed their work in three months, gaining the title "ninety-day wonders," a title given by regular army men and the general public.

Tom Powell had a strong feeling for the military, much of which came from the service of his grandfathers in the Civil War. On Sunday afternoons in his youth, he would hear stories of that war from elderly Confederate veterans who lived in Warren County. Those personal stories were the primary way Tom and his young friends could learn about the war, and they listened eagerly and in awe of what those veterans had endured and accomplished.

After his ninety days of training, Tom left college for duty at an army base in Plattsburg, New York, a beautiful spot on the Hudson River. He served as a rifle instructor while attached to the military training program at nearby Syracuse University. He was not there long before the war ended on November 11, 1918, and he was discharged in December. Tom Powell returned to Elon College at the age of eighteen not only as a military veteran but as an officer as well. When he left the army he did not lose his interest in the military. In fact, he remained an officer in the reserves, attaining the rank of captain before retiring eleven years later.

Back at school he applied himself to his studies and graduated, ready for a place in the working world. During his time at Elon he had attracted the attention of administration and faculty because of his work ethic and his general excellence in his studies. As a result, the college offered him a job as an instructor in geology and botany. The young graduate accepted the position with the enthusiasm he had shown in his studies and his military service.

As he went about developing his teaching program, he did considerable laboratory work, and it soon became obvious that he needed an assistant for that work to be more effective. He found that assistant in the person of Sophia Maude Sharpe, a student from the Bellemont community in southern Alamance County. She was an outstanding student leader and also a good athlete, starring in tennis and basketball. But most important was her interest in the sciences, particularly biology and chemistry, and she was chosen for the lab position. Pretty soon the word was around campus that Tom Powell had a very sharp laboratory assistant. The two shared a good working relationship that grew into a strong personal attraction. They were married in 1922.

While teaching, Powell continued his own education by driving to Chapel Hill and Durham on nights and weekends to expand his knowledge of the sciences. He earned a master's degree in geology and botany from UNC in 1923 and a year later earned the rank of professor at Elon College. In 1930 he received his PhD from Duke University. At that time he was teaching at Elon College and running a growing business while studying for his graduate degree.

During those early years he and his wife, Maude, had a daughter, Sophia, born in 1925. Maude looked after their daughter while continuing work as a laboratory assistant, counting specimens and performing other jobs in support of her husband as he continued his studies. Her support and assistance during those years were not unnoticed. At graduation in 1930 a Duke official said he did not know who deserved the PhD more—Tom Powell or Maude.

While all this was going on, Tom continued his teaching duties, striving always to make the work more meaningful for his students. In his early years of teaching, he realized that he really did not have the supplies that he needed in his laboratory to give students the best possible learning experience. As he looked around, he realized this was true at most other colleges and universities around the nation. There had to be a better way, he believed, so he went in search of it.

In 1927 he joined with a teaching colleague at Elon College and formed Carolina Biological Supply Co. just east of the college campus. It did not take long to realize that the needs he saw were real, and the company filled those needs by providing biological specimens and materials for classrooms all across the nation. While there was a need for the materials that Carolina Biological supplied, the timing for beginning the company certainly could have been better. Just as the company was getting off the ground, the greatest economic depression in the history of the nation struck with unimaginable severity. Tom Powell had to continue to teach while working at the company at nights and on weekends and finishing his own education.

The college also felt major hardships from the Depression, and in fact there was difficulty in meeting the payroll for the faculty. At one point the college went for four months without being able to pay the professors and staff members.

While Tom Powell faced that situation, his wife was able to continue her job teaching at Elon College High School. One of the things that was certain in the Depression was payment to public school teachers by the state of North Carolina. Maude sacrificed many of the extras in life to allow her husband to make Carolina Biological succeed. With her check from the state, the little family was able to make it through those difficult years.

Carolina Biological was growing more successful every day, but the college's

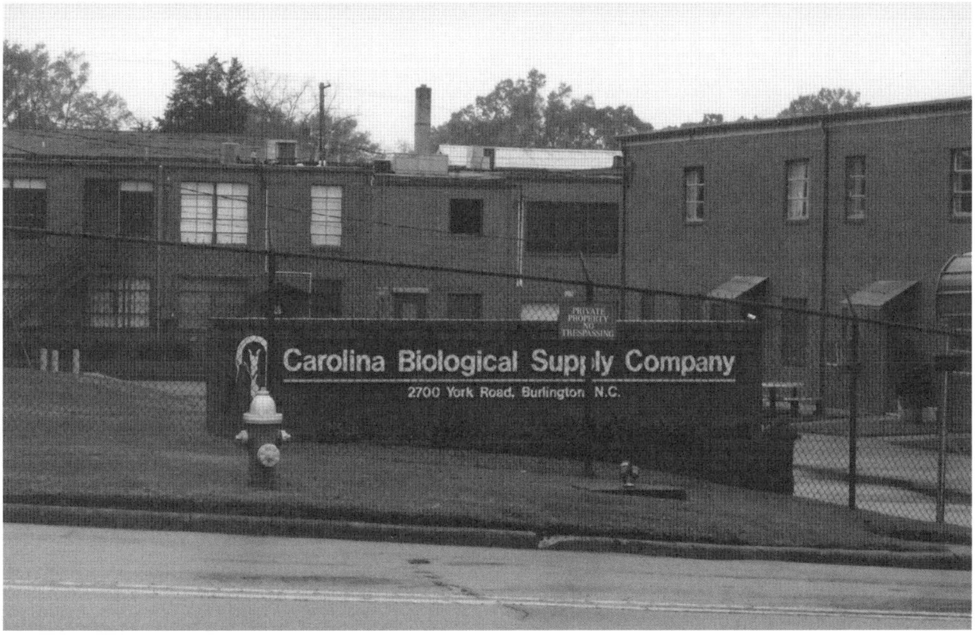

Carolina Biological Supply Co. in Burlington, NC

finances continued to struggle. At that point, Tom left the classrooms of Elon College and devoted his attention to managing Carolina Biological.

Along the way he had become a member of the North Carolina Academy of Science in 1921, and he also worked to benefit educational programs both on the local and state levels. He was a member of the Alamance County Board of Education for twenty-seven years, from 1934 to 1961. He was vice president of the North Carolina School Board Association in 1938 and 1939, and president of that group from 1943 to 1945. He also served on a number of other community and state boards over the years.

The Powell family grew in 1936 when Thomas Edward Powell III was born, and two years later came twin sons—John Sharpe Powell and James Bobbitt Powell.

Sadness visited the family in 1944, however, when Maude Sharpe Powell died of breast cancer. Daughter Sophia was graduating from Duke University that year, but Edward was only seven and the twins were five. It was a difficult time for the family, and they faced an uncertain future with the loss of their mother.

At that time, Dr. Powell's sister, Caroline E. Powell, agreed to come to Elon College and help the family. She was then a teacher at Needham Broughton High School in Raleigh, but she agreed to move into her brother's home and help care for the three young children. That arrangement quickly expanded as Caroline began to help her brother in the business as well as caring for the children. "Miss Caroline" developed the marketing plan for the company's mail order business, and she became responsible for all the company's accounts receivable.

Even during World War II, the company continued its growth. In January 1945 Carolina Biological opened a subsidiary, Waubun Laboratories, in Schriever, Louisiana. That operation was established for the collection of specimens in the bayous of Louisiana as well as preparations of skeletons in the winter months.

Carolina Biological Supply Company built a highly favorable reputation by providing superior products delivered efficiently and on time. It was absolutely necessary for classroom specimens and supplies to reach the classrooms on Monday morning for use that day. To do that, CBSC paid overtime to employees to work on a regular basis until noon on Saturday, and some worked all day to make sure the deliveries were accurate and on time.

A typical business day at the company began with opening the mail first thing in the morning. Each order was stamped with a number, and an order was generated with an acknowledgment sent out that same day. Before the close of business on a given day, every department was to have received the new orders, and Caroline Powell took checks downtown to the bank.

In 1945 Tom Powell married Annabelle Council, and in the years that followed they had three sons and a daughter: Bill, Joe, Sam, and Beth.

The years of the 1940s and 1950s were good for Carolina Biological, and its business continued to enjoy a slow but certain growth. During that period and for many years after, the United States was locked in the Cold War with the Soviet Union. A part of that was competition in scientific development, especially in space. As a result, the federal government began pumping money into scientific education in general, and Carolina Biological enjoyed a major surge in growth.

Three Brothers Eye the Future

Also during those years, Ed, John, and Jim were growing up in the scientific business environment in the Powell family. They were making their own preparations for their futures in that environment. Ed and Jim entered medical school at Duke University, and John was in law school at the same institution.

Each of the three young men was looking to the time he would move into the family enterprise, but each looked at different areas of the business. It was also Tom Powell's plan for those sons to follow in the business in the years ahead.

All three had attended Virginia Military Institute and went on to Duke University for graduate work. The three had grown up in a family that expected hard work and highly valued a good education. Their parents were teachers, and all four of their aunts were educators as well. Their parents worked hard and made sacrifices to assure the success of their business.

Dr. Powell expected that same work ethic from his sons. As a teenager, Jim Powell remembers working at Waubun Laboratories for Carolina Biological. It was hard work, which is what his father expected. He wanted his sons to have goals in life, and he wanted them to earn their PhDs in biological sciences and eventually return to work at Carolina Biological Supply Co. It was a good plan, at least in Dr. Powell's mind.

But the sons had gained much from growing up in a hard-working and scientifically oriented family. They also had learned to think for themselves. Each liked the idea of a career in science, but they were uncertain as to the direction they wanted to take. Ed and Jim were attracted to medicine, which led them to Duke University Medical School. John, however, had his eye on business law, so he received his Duke degree in law.

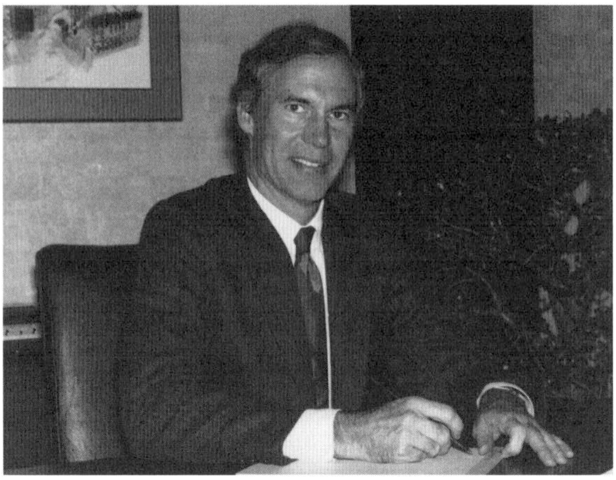

Dr. James B. Powell

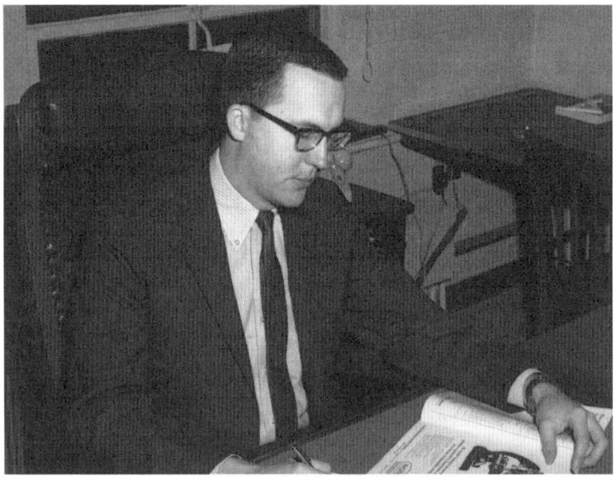

John Powell

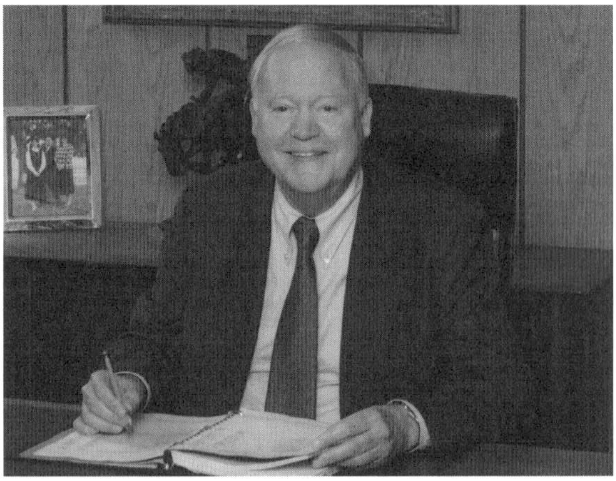

Dr. T. E. Powell III

CHAPTER TWO

Biomedical Laboratories Is Formed

EVENTUALLY THE THREE BROTHERS decided to form their own company, a medical testing laboratory they named Biomedical Laboratories. They saw this laboratory as filling the needs that Jim had found while in his studies at Duke. The lab could cut down tremendously on the time required to get lab results and make the entire testing system more efficient.

The three young men who conceived of this idea had considerable technical knowledge but little business training in the academic sense. However, they had plenty of practical experience, and they could draw on the support and knowledge of their father, the first of the Powell entrepreneurs. The only thing the Powell brothers had resembling a business plan was a collection of technical documents and financial agreements relating to the company's funding. Despite the lack of a business plan, the three young men relied on specific technical knowledge and general business experience, including in sales and marketing, to help them launch Biomedical Laboratories. Each was well prepared in those areas.

Ed provided vital services in the early days of Biomedical Laboratories, assisting with purchases and interfacing with Carolina Biological. Ed had been the first to enter Duke, and he was quite successful as an understudy to Dr. Wayne Rundles, who was head of hematology at the university. Dr. Rundles was highly impressed with Ed and became a mentor to him, pointing him to a possible career in academic medicine. Ed was chosen to be a member of the first class of the MD/PhD program at Duke, a program that has a national reputation as it continues today.

Ed worked for five years with Dr. Keith Porter at Harvard University in the study of cellular biology. Dr. Porter was internationally recognized for studies of cells using the electron microscope, which was much more powerful than any microscopes previously in use. The first electron microscope was built by the Siemens AG Corporation in Nazi-dominated Germany in the 1930s. This specialized technology was later incorporated into various lines offered by Carolina Biological.

After leaving Harvard, Ed served three years at the National Institutes of Health (NIH) in the Washington, DC, area. He then returned to North Carolina to become president of the family business, and today he continues as majority owner and chairman of Carolina Biological Supply Co.

Jim began at Walter Reed Army Institute of Research in Washington in 1969 and also served as president and medical director of Biomedical Laboratories, visiting on weekends. He did that through the first three years of the young company's existence while also serving on its board of directors.

Following graduation from Duke, John served the required years of military service just as the United States was increasing its presence in Vietnam. He entered the army as a first lieutenant in artillery at Fort Sill, Oklahoma. After his military duty, John entered Tulane University and obtained his MBA. He then returned to Carolina Biological and later played a major role in the development of financial and business functions at Biomedical Laboratories. When Jim decided to enter Duke Medical School, he found the admission process much easier because of the outstanding reputation held there by his brother Ed, who had entered three years earlier. Jim was not excited about a career in biology or at Carolina Biological. He was more interested in combining medicine and business, but he had not figured out how to do that early in his education journey. But one day it came to him as a senior medical student while talking to his brother Ed. It was a moment of epiphany, he recalls, when he learned that pathologists were the specialists who ran medical testing laboratories.

That was it. Then he remembered how difficult it was to get proper medical testing accomplished. He thought of the time it took in medical school to send tests to the West Coast and the problems that created. He said the idea crystallized in his mind "like a flash." From that point, Biomedical Laboratories began to take shape, one step on a journey that eventually would help give birth to LabCorp in later years.

With the decision to take this path, there also came the realities the company would face along the way.

Starting a laboratory from scratch required a qualified director, and that requirement would add another five years for a newly minted physician after his four years in medical school. Those five years would allow the director to sit for the board exams to qualify as an anatomical and clinical pathologist. Even when that was done, there was the realization that money would be tight, and the group could not go out and hire a qualified pathologist in the open market. Pathologists were well compensated at the time, and in addition, the pathology community was not excited about formation of a commercial laboratory. The idea was considered a radical venture that had not been done before on any scale.

With that picture hanging over the process, Jim immediately applied to the pathology department at Duke to begin his postgraduate work as an intern in that department. He had a five-year journey ahead of him to become board certified as a pathologist, but he was becoming part of an outstanding program at Duke. Dr. Thomas Kinney had recently succeeded Dr. Wiley Forbus as chair of the pathology department there, and he was held in high regard throughout the field.

Jim enjoyed his years at Duke, but he was also anxious to receive training elsewhere. Dr. Kinney called some of his friends around the nation and found a spot for Jim at New York Hospital / Cornell Medical Center in New York City. He had two good years there in anatomical pathology and cytology training. He spent an additional two years at Englewood Hospital in New Jersey with Dr. S. Raymond Gambino, which was a stroke of good fortune for Jim Powell. Dr. Gambino was widely recognized as a national leader in clinical chemistry. Dr. Gambino was already aware of the reputation of Carolina Biological Supply Co. when he interviewed the young candidate for study with him. Jim spent his fourth and fifth years of residency training in pathology with Dr. Gambino, having already completed three years in anatomic pathology at Duke and Cornell.

At Englewood, Jim met a young man who was working as a medical technologist there. Ernie Knesel and Jim became friends, often meeting and talking in the hallways or at coffee breaks. Knesel said, "I got to know him in the clinical chemistry laboratory." Powell was a resident; Knesel, a laboratory technologist. Knesel remembers that "we respected and enjoyed each other," and a good friendship developed. They also shared a common interest: starting an independent clinical laboratory in the South.

Knesel was born in New Orleans and had lived in Atlanta before his family moved to New Jersey. His father was in shipping with Sea Train Lines, the first company to ship railroad boxcars on oceangoing ships.

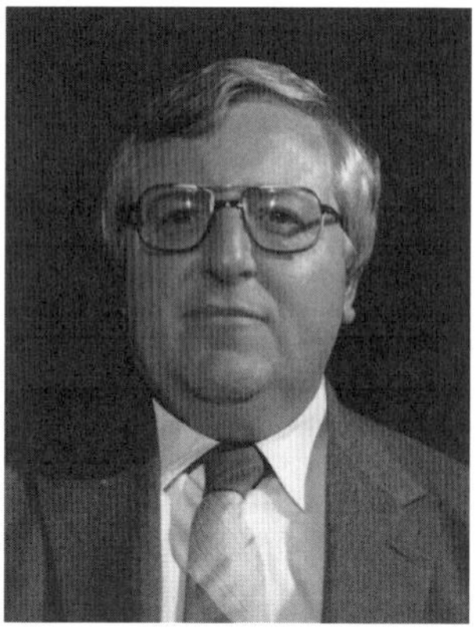

Ernie Knesel

Ernie Knesel had one year of college in Savannah and then went to Fairleigh-Dickenson when his family moved north. He graduated there and later received his master's degree in that university's dentistry biomedical program.

Knesel was married while at Englewood, and he and his wife, Lynn, worked side by side, as she was a laboratory technologist as well.

When Powell and Knesel were at Englewood Hospital, another resident had some ambitions similar to their own—Paul Brown. Brown later created MetPath Laboratories, and Knesel said, "We saw MetPath started. It ignited Jim's interest. He wanted to do something in Burlington." That was when the two friends began talking seriously about creating a laboratory. Knesel said the two decided, "If Brown could do it, we could do it."

Laboratory facilities were almost nonexistent at the time. "There was a lab in Oregon, but it was cheap and not so good," Knesel said. "We could do it better." And as Knesel also said, "I wanted to go back South."

When Powell said he wanted to create the lab, Knesel was absolutely interested. "It was an opportunity to operate our own lab under Jim."

Jim had exposure at Englewood to the very latest in lab equipment. Dr. Gambino had received what was called an SMA (sequential multiple analyzer) 12/60, a machine produced by Technicon that revolutionized laboratory procedures. It was the first true automation in the clinical laboratory. Dr. Gambino allowed Jim to participate in one of the first training sessions for the SMA 12/60, and Jim became one of the most knowledgeable people in the nation about that equipment. The SMA 12/60 combined many single-channel analyzers into one machine. It was capable of performing twelve tests per minute on one single sample of blood serum, and it produced a chart of those results that could be placed directly into a patient's medical records.

Technicon had worked for a number of years in laboratory automation before developing the SMA 12/60. The company first developed an automated tissue processor to prepare tissue to be cut and prepared as microscopic slides. The company later developed a system of single-channel analyzers that made it possible to run a specific test on multiple samples. For instance, it was possible to run 150 blood glucose analyses on different samples and to accomplish the batch of tests at a rate of approximately one test per minute.

Later a double-channel analyzer was developed to make it possible to run two tests at one time on one instrument. Technicon later created the Sequential Multiple Analysis Computerized analyzer that would greatly increase the ability of Biomedical Laboratories to better serve their customers when the company was up and running.

According to Jim Powell, the automated analyzer and the beginnings of more advanced telecommunications were setting the stage for large automated clinical laboratories across the nation. He trained for three months on the 12/60 before going to Washington, DC, for his three-year tour with the military.

Powell and Knesel continued their talks and saw great potential for an entirely new business that delivered highly automated laboratory analyses in quick fashion. In fact, they spent a great deal of time developing a list of every piece of equipment they would need.

It was 1969 by then, and the idea of a laboratory in Burlington was beginning to become more clear. A good facility was needed, along with financing. Funds were needed to purchase a 12/60 analyzer and other lab equipment, as well as for hiring personnel. The Powell brothers and Knesel had no resources of which to speak, and there was little possibility of obtaining help from a bank.

Knesel remembers that the three brothers had not told their father about their plans.

The First Day at Work

But on June 2, 1969, Knesel went to work, and his location was at the Carolina Biological Supply Co. site. He happened to be working outside Ed Powell's office, and someone asked him, "Who are you?"

He said he was waiting to see Dr. Powell, and at that point Dr. Thomas Powell Jr. learned that his sons were getting the lab business started quickly. He was surprised, but by day's end he was on board with the idea, according to Knesel.

Knesel said that was the day that the business venture became known to everyone, and the brothers turned to their father for help. That first day on the job also happened to be the first wedding anniversary for Ernie and his wife, Lynn.

All the equipment that Jim Powell and Ernie Knesel had listed back in New Jersey as needed had been ordered in advance. It was not ordered through CBS but other companies. But when Dr. Thomas Powell got involved, he had them cancel the orders and everything was reordered through Carolina Biological. Knesel said Dr. Powell said he could get a better deal—and he did.

Ron Sturgill was working with American Hospital Supply Corp. in Charlotte at that time. "I had my first contact with the lab in Burlington." He had received orders for laboratory equipment from Englewood Hospital in New Jersey. But it was not long before he received instructions to ignore those orders and that the supplies were being purchased by Carolina Biological Supply Co. in Burlington, North Carolina. Sturgill did not know it then, but one day he would be a part of that new laboratory in Burlington.

The idea began to form between the Powells and Knesel that it would be good to wait until Jim had completed his military service before launching the new lab. The elder Dr. Powell initially felt strongly about this.

The major competitor in the eyes of the Powell group was National Health Laboratories in Arlington, Virginia. While at Walter Reed, Jim had an opportunity to visit that lab—dressed in his military uniform. People at the lab must have assumed he was a potential customer, and they shared information freely, including plans to open a laboratory in central North Carolina in the near future.

Paul Brown, the pathology resident in the Gambino program in New Jersey, was also working to get his laboratory up and running in New Jersey in the spring of 1969. Brown started Metropolitan Pathology Laboratory, Inc. in New York and then the company changed its name to MetPath, Inc. and later to Quest Diagnostic Incorporated, today LabCorp's major national competitor. In fact, in 2015, LabCorp was number one in the nation, and Quest was number two.

All this activity by future competitors made Jim Powell feel the urgency to move and not wait until he was out of the army in three years. But others were not so sure. The Powell group had these considerations for the startup date for their own laboratory. They could not agree during a weekend meeting in the spring of 1969, when Jim came home from Washington. They met Friday and Saturday but could reach no plan. Jim had to leave on Sunday afternoon, but that morning he visited his father and laid out a plan for the immediate launch of the company. The elder Powell finally relented that morning to start immediately. They would occupy part of the old Alamance General Hospital, already owned by Carolina Biological. The elder Dr. Powell had purchased the old hospital site with no particular use in mind. He thought perhaps it might be useful as more laboratory space for Carolina Biological, but it proved to be just the right facility at just the right time for Biomedical Laboratories to lease in 1969.

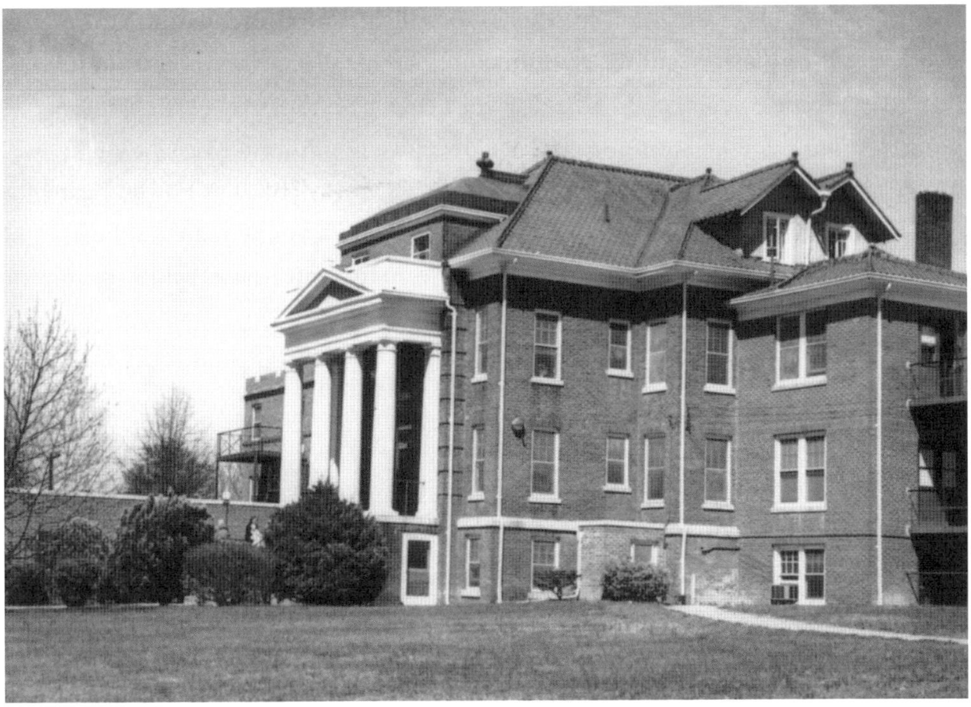

Alamance General Hospital, Burlington, NC

The brothers would lease the property, and each would contribute approximately twenty-five thousand dollars of his own money, and the elder Powell would loan them sixty thousand dollars. Later an agreement was reached with Wachovia Bank for financing, but the brothers had to pledge their houses in Burlington as collateral.

A key part of Jim's plan was to bring Ernie Knesel to Burlington to run the laboratory, with Jim coming from Washington every weekend he could get off from the army. When presenting this part of the idea, there was no mention of the fact that Knesel was a very young man with absolutely no experience in management. He was twenty-three years old. Knesel remembers one of the brothers, John, asking at the time, "You want me to invest in a company headed by a twenty-three-year-old?" Actually, none of the founders had any management experience beyond their training at VMI to be army officers.

Surprisingly, the elder Powell and the others agreed to Jim's plan, and the wheels started to turn for an opening at the earliest possible date. It indeed was surprising that Dr. Thomas Powell Jr. had changed his mind, and to this day no one is certain why he did so. Justifying his earlier purchase of the old hospital may have been a factor, as well as his desire to see his sons launch their careers and to utilize the expensive educations that he had totally funded for them. Whatever his reason, it was a timely move.

Knesel developed a strong respect for the elder Dr. Powell. Knesel remembered one occasion when he requisitioned some chairs from CBS. Dr. Powell heard the request and asked, "Why do you want chairs? You are a young man and need to be working, not sitting down." It was said, of course, in fun, but Knesel said it was typical of the elder Powell.

The First Sample Is Tested

The first sample tested in the laboratory on its first day of operations in October 1969 was a blood sample from Dr. Thomas E. Powell Jr. Knesel said that sample was sealed in plastic, and it remains as a reminder of the launching of the company.

Knesel also said that, on the first day, Dr. Ed Powell went to his own personal physician and was tested and brought the sample to the lab for analysis. He asked others in the lab to go and do the same thing.

When operations began, Knesel and his wife worked together. "She was hourly and got time and a half, but I was the overall supervisor," and he did enjoy the extra pay for extra work. Knesel also did some selling, and in fact did whatever was needed at a particular time. He and his wife were the first two employees of the new company.

In the first three years, Knesel ran the operations. "I reported to Ed, and Jim came on weekends [from his military duties] to kick the tires.... We got good support from Ed Powell," he remembers. "He even moved people over from Carolina Biological Supply." Janice Ray was one of them, coming on as a secretary in the new operation. She stayed with the company through all the changes and went on to be an administrative assistant to Tom Mac Mahon, when he was president and CEO of LabCorp. Janice Ray is still at LabCorp almost fifty years later.

John Kinney also came at that time from CBSC. He ran the office and ran updates and did some sales. "He was a specialist in developing special forms," Knesel explains, and some of them are still in use today. He went on to operate his own specialized printing company for business forms for many years.

Two weeks before the first specimen was tested, National Health Laboratories became the first automated commercial laboratory in North Carolina by opening an operation in Greensboro, a scant thirty miles from Burlington.

An immediate race began between the two, with National Health concentrating on western North Carolina and Biomedical concentrating on the east. Later National Health moved into Baptist Hospital in Winston-Salem.

Biomedical Laboratories quickly acquired clients, and the future looked exciting. It was also clear that had there been a delay of three years, the success of the new company would have been adversely impacted and may not, in fact, have been possible at all. In moving as quickly as they did, the Biomedical founders learned the truth of an old adage: Timing is everything.

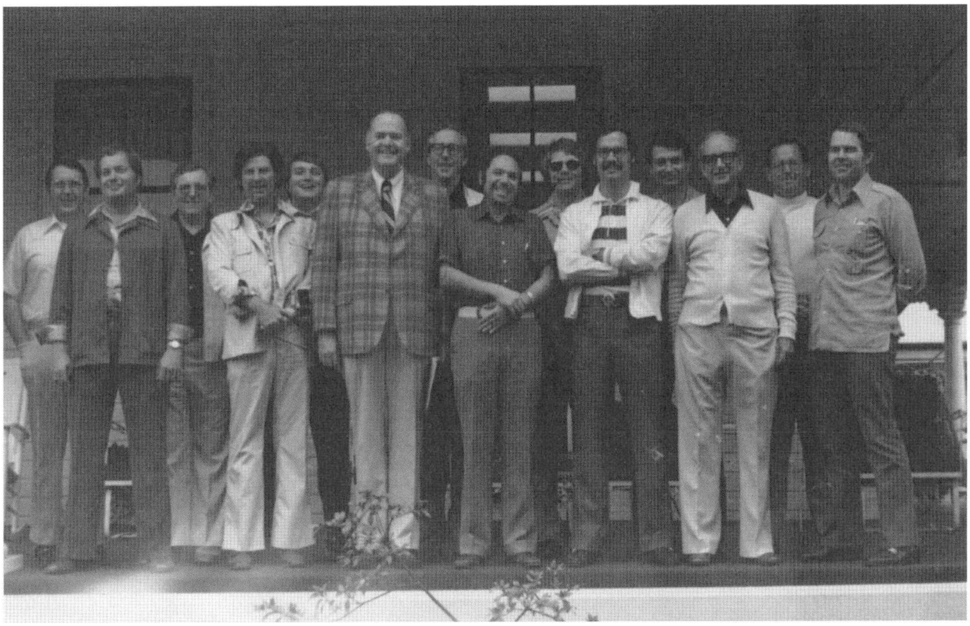

Early management team for Biomedical Laboratories—left to right, Bob Harrington, Wayne Kempff, Poe Jenrette, Jim Folks, Ed Powell, John Powell, Boris Datnow, Bill Irwin, Jim Powell, Paul Hoffner, Hinton Rountree, Elmer Walker and Jim Creech

CHAPTER THREE

Business Practices at Biomedical Laboratories

WHEN BIOMEDICAL LABORATORIES began operations, its owners did not have to look very far for business practices that made the company stand apart from its competitors. They looked to Carolina Biological Supply Co. and Dr. Thomas E. Powell Jr.

Dr. Powell had realized that prompt service was vital to satisfying the needs of his customers. Therefore, he established a workweek of forty-four hours for employees at Carolina Biological. They worked the regular forty-hour week and then another four hours on Saturday morning with overtime pay. This allowed Carolina to get specimens and supplies in the mail on Saturday afternoon in time for classroom activities on Monday morning. Other suppliers could not, or would not, go to those lengths. As a result, CBSC soon had the reputation as the best company for timely service in the biological supply industry.

Biomedical Laboratories adopted that same workweek with Saturday hours, and its reputation for service was quickly established. The company also adapted CBS's system of daily reports, a system that Dr. Thomas Powell learned while in the military. The first daily report from October 6, 1969, showed revenues of forty-five dollars for the first day of operations.

Other valuable business advice came from Robert Townsend's bestsellers, *Up the Organization in 1970* and *Further Up the Organization* in the early 1980s. Townsend gained fame for bringing the Avis rental car company out of financial troubles. He had a no-nonsense approach to running a large company that was not dominated by corporate politics or favoritisms. He called this "participative management." Biomedical adopted many of his practices, and some were quite simple. For instance, there were no private parking spaces—for anyone, including executives. Parking was on a first-come, first-served basis. That rule survived for many years. There was also the idea of sharing ownership with employees. A profit-sharing plan was put into effect, as were an employee stock ownership plan and equity awards to key employees.

Townsend was opposed to the idea of calling on hired consultants for key decisions—consultants who might know little about the operations. He recommended calling on employees for their input. Townsend also said no to long meetings, alcohol at business luncheons, nepotism, and "big wheels in little companies."

Biomedical Laboratories' initial plan of operations was rather simple. Company couriers drove to medical offices in the area—Burlington, Greensboro, and High Point—to pick up specimens and return them to the laboratory where they were analyzed overnight. The next day the reports were returned to the doctors and new specimens were picked up. This twenty-four-hour service was revolutionary in the lab business and a key to the success of the operations from day one.

Jim Powell addressed this service in an article in 1982. He said that what his company had done was essentially to take lab tests to the practicing physician, while in the past those tests were available only in research centers. That gave the small-town North Carolina physician the same access to any laboratory test that a doctor at Duke Medical Center had. Powell added that his company could probably get the results back more quickly.

The first facility the young company occupied was a good fit for its operations. The building in 1916 had been the first major hospital built in Alamance County. Dr. Rainey Parker was a general practitioner who operated the hospital as Rainey Hospital until 1922, when he was joined by Dr. R. E. Brooks. Dr. Parker later left, and Dr. George Carrington joined Dr. Brooks in 1927. The two would have a long partnership. In 1937 the facility became known as Alamance General Hospital and had its first board of directors. It was expanded in 1949 to sixty-four beds.

A second hospital, Alamance County Hospital, was opened in 1951, and Alamance General continued for another ten years. At that time Memorial Hospital opened, replacing Alamance General. Dr. Carrington continued operating in the clinic portion at the old location for a few more years.

Celo Faucette was one of the first people hired by the new company. He was one of the first drivers who made the daily trips to pick up specimens.

"There were three of us at first, and we tried to see who could get the most" specimens. There was a lot of competition among them. When they hit one hundred, it was a big event, he said.

The three were driving Ford Cortinas, and Faucette remembers that when they came to a big hill, "we would have to use the passing gear" to get up that hill. Later another driver was added, along with a Volkswagen that had air-conditioning. "The four of us would rotate" so that each driver had air-conditioning once every four weeks.

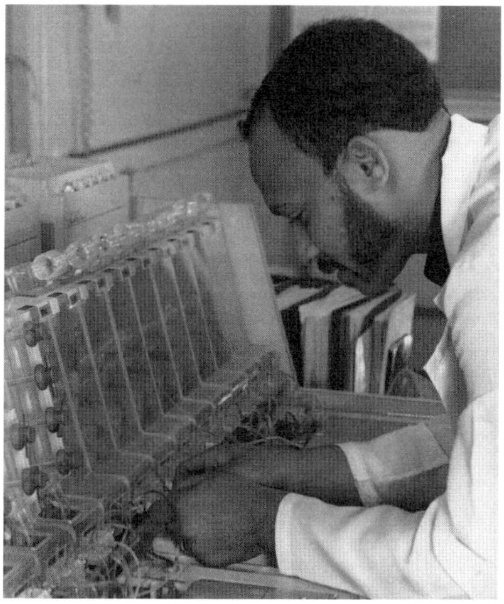
Celo Faucette

They wrote their reports by hand, Faucette said, and there was a lot more to the job than just making sales and picking up specimens. "We did whatever we had to do to make the company successful." He remembers that Ernie Knesel and his wife painted the interior of the hospital area they were using as a lab.

Faucette remembers that they recycled anything usable, including labels on the specimens. If one was not used, it would be taken off and put on another, something that would not be allowed today. And no one used the elevator. It never worked properly.

Faucette also remembers that there was fun along the way. When a new person came in the lab, "We would put apple juice in a urine container and drink it" for their benefit. He said those new people wondered what they were getting into.

In 1975 Faucette transferred to Memphis, where he was lab manager, and then he spent some years in the District of Columbia in sales, then in Research Triangle Park, then in Atlanta, then back to RTP, and finally back to Burlington as facilities manager. He retired in 2005.

As Faucette reflected on his career, he stated his appreciation for Dr. Jim Powell and all the Powell family. It was a most enjoyable situation, he said, like a big family working together. "We had a good opportunity to grow, and most of us stayed on." He said working there made it possible to have a good life, a good home, and good opportunities for his family. Since retirement, Faucette has moved into the political field and in 2016 was serving as mayor pro tem of the city of Burlington.

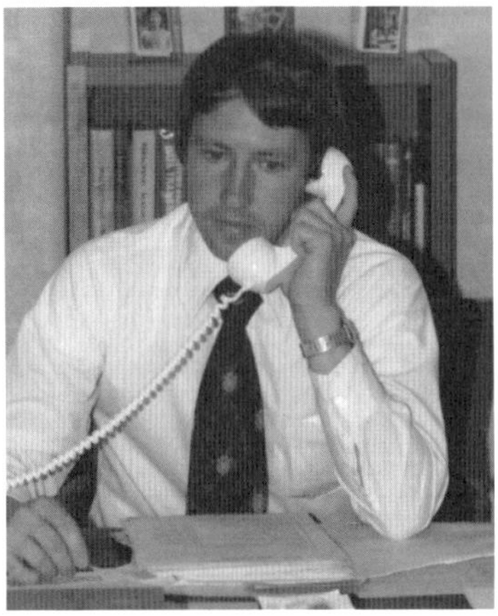

Jesse Long

It is hard to imagine in the computerized world of the twenty-first century that there were no computers in use in the early days of Biomedical Laboratories. Jesse Long remembers that time well, and he recalls how the company functioned with systems that are seen today as unbelievably primitive.

Long was one of the early employees of the new company, joining the firm in January 1970. He had just completed four years with the air force in security services. When he joined Biomedical Laboratories he did not realize it, but that background would serve him well. He was hired by Dr. Ed Powell as Dr. Jim Powell was still in the military.

Long had a spot on the third shift in the early years, working as part of the continuing process that brought samples in for testing, the testing itself, the preparation of reports, and the return of the report to the doctor or hospital where it had originated.

At that time, Long explained, service representatives picked up samples during the day from the customers and brought them to the laboratory. The night shift ran the tests. Then on an IBM Selectric typewriter, someone prepared the report on forms that included several copies. The representatives who picked up the samples returned the reports the next day as they picked up new samples.

Long said it fell to the third shift to read the reports the second shift made. They had to check to be sure that everything was accurate, and he said that an MD on the staff, Dr. Betty Beck, taught him how to do that. After some time, Long laughed and said that finally, "A computer replaced me." But Long moved on to other duties and remained with the company for twenty-eight years.

He said the early procedure of picking up, testing, and returning reports worked well while the area of service was small. As the area served began to grow, the company had to rely on mail or other methods, one of which was Piedmont Airlines. Results were flown to an office in another area, and a representative there took them to the customers.

Long said doctors wanted their reports early in the morning before they made rounds, and mail or driving was taking too long. To solve that problem, the company turned to the teletype. As the samples were tested, reports were written during the night and put out early the next morning by teletype to the doctors or hospitals.

"It was a very competitive business," Long said. "We had to get the reports out early or someone else got the business."

There was a huge cost in using the telephone lines, and sometimes they were not all that reliable, he said. Paper tapes were a key part of the teletype operation, and Long said the company found innovative ways to get all the information needed onto that tape. He said his military work in encryption came in handy as ways had to be devised to keep the information on the tapes safe.

Ernie Knesel said Biomedical Laboratories was the first lab in the country to use remote reporting by teletype. It was typical of the company, he said, to take such innovative steps.

"Innovation was a big strength of the company. We did what we had to do to beat the competition," he said, repeating a phrase several others in the company have used over the years.

Long said that as the company moved along with this system, they developed their own printers, which were sent to customers all over the country to improve the process. He said there must have been ten thousand of those printers in use at one time. The entire process was highly time-sensitive, and ways were constantly sought to find ways to improve the speed element.

To this day, Long has a reminder of that era on his desk—a little memento: a piece of that paper tape molded in Plexiglas from Dr. Jim Powell with the date March 23, 1983.

It was not long, however, until computers became vital to Biomedical operations.

Centralized Computer System Vital

A centralized computer approach for the entire company was developed in the early years. Obviously the approach was a good one, as LabCorp has continued using much of the original software from Biomedical Laboratories to this day.

Early financial functions were performed on software written by the Biomedical information system staff for an IBM system. Actually that software was run first on a contractual basis on the IBM computer at Glen Raven Mills. Later an IBM System 3 was installed in the Rainey building.

The early computers at the old General Hospital site, Long said, were quite big and used large boards that contained the information needed for test information. Along about 1980, he remembered, the computers were moved to the new York Court location. As time passed, new laboratories were built or acquired, and they were brought on line with the central computer in Burlington. Eventually the computer function was moved to a facility in the Research Triangle, when the lab became Roche Biomedical Laboratories.

Biomedical Laboratories' unique computer approach provided better customer service and better quality control, and it also laid the framework for the formation of LabCorp, now the largest laboratory operation in the world.

Jesse Long retired after twenty-eight years and then went on to a second career of sixteen years with Alamance Regional Medical Center in communications. His words about speed in the testing process and the tremendous pressure from competition were echoed by another longtime employee of the company.

Bill Cox spent thirty-two years in the operation before his retirement, much of that time in sales. Cox was a college student working in a stereo store when he became friends with Paul Hoffner, a frequent customer in the store. Hoffner was a vice president with Biomedical Laboratories who lived in Gibsonville, North Carolina. Cox talked a few times with Hoffner about where he might get a job after college, and Hoffner set him up for an interview at a South Carolina location of the company. Cox landed the job in 1975 and began a career that took him to a high position in sales management, heading up the South Atlantic Region and the Hospital Division in that region.

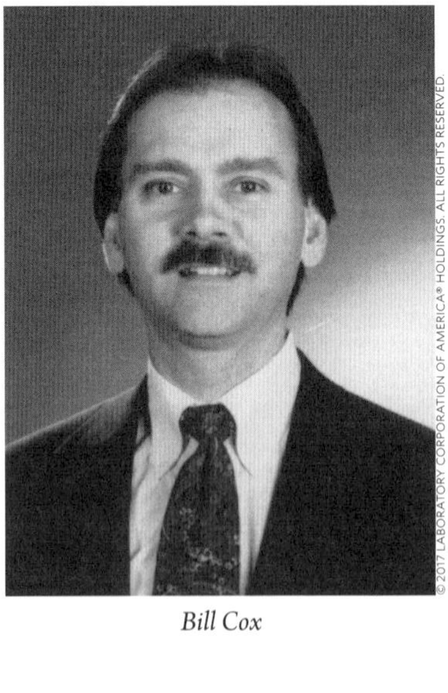

Bill Cox

Selling laboratory testing was quite different from selling other goods and services to doctors and hospitals. Patients visiting medical clinics often see a person with a large case on wheels walking by. That person is obviously a sales representative for a pharmaceutical company. The salesperson tells the doctor what the new drug will do and leaves samples for the doctor's use. Then the doctor can see the results. Selling a medical test is not only an entirely different thing, but it can sometimes be quite difficult.

Cox said, "We were selling a promise of a future service—a promise to pick up samples, do a test, and return a good product in a timely way. And what we had to sell was still evolving," he said. New tests were being added all the time.

"Our process was valuable to the doctor. It was so much better than what they already had," he said. And what the doctors already had were local hospitals.

Cox was selling the promise of overnight service, and it was "so less expensive." He said the salespeople would go into a town and find where the doctors were and make their calls. Hospitals were not at all happy about this invasion and the loss of testing revenue.

As time passed, however, more labs were brought into the Biomedical Laboratories family and more services were added. Cox said that hospitals then found it beneficial to send their tests to the company as well. Tests also became far more technical and sophisticated, and sales personnel found that they had to offer something beyond the basics. Training became a vital part of sales, as the personnel had to be able to explain a test in technical detail in order to operate effectively to the customer's satisfaction.

Cox, who worked in Columbia, South Carolina; Memphis, Tennessee; and finally Raleigh, North Carolina, remembers from his days in operations the teletype machines that Jesse Long described.

Those teletypes got results, Cox remembers, but they were time-consuming. "We had to put the name of the patient, the doctor, and the test on each one," he said. In 1975 or so, the company moved over to the Univac 9000 computer, which allowed the entries to be made at a terminal.

Savannah, Georgia, was one of the early sites testing that computer, he said. He was working in Columbia, South Carolina, at the time, and on one occasion he was called temporarily to Savannah.

"I was working there as a backup courier," and when he was no longer needed, "I left for Columbia." Then it was decided that Savannah would go live with the computer that night, and "they wanted me to stay." But those working with the computer were told he was already gone. The word was to "get him back."

Communications, of course, were far from what they are today. There were no cell phones, no easy way to contact him on the highway. Cox said he was about halfway to Columbia when he was pulled by a highway patrolman.

"Scared the fool out of me," he said. He was twenty-three years old and had never been stopped and did not know what to expect.

The officer told him there was an emergency in Savannah and his presence was needed. Those in Savannah had called the Highway Patrol to find Cox. He went to the patrol station, made a call, and then returned to Savannah.

Cox said logistics was one of the major keys to the success of early operations at Biomed.

"There was a real sense of urgency about getting tests [reports] back on time. If the plane did not fly, we drove four hours to make the delivery. We did basic things to get them there on time. We were not good at first and had to learn."

"We Did Whatever Had to Be Done"

Simply put, Cox said, "we did whatever had to be done" to finish tasks on time.

Neither Cox nor Long was educated for work in a laboratory testing company, nor did either have any experience in the field. Long came from the air force, and Cox came out of college via a stereo shop. But both had long and successful careers with LabCorp and its predecessors, and both rose to positions of major importance in the company.

That was not unusual. A number of employees have similar stories during the company's history. Another example of that success is Cheryl Van Vorous.

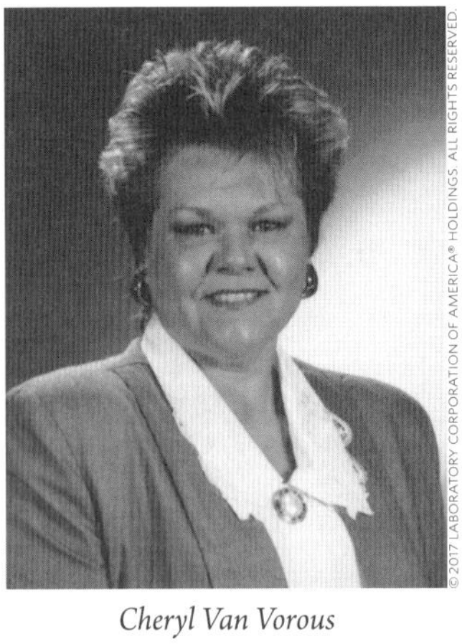

Cheryl Van Vorous

"I went in October 1, 1973, at twenty-three years old and out June 30, 2010, at sixty years old," she said. And she went in as a secretary and came out as a vice president. She handled relations with the pathologists who worked for the company.

Van Vorous started in the sales department, and after a short time she was moved to accounting. It was something in which she was simply not interested. She manually calculated the compensation for the early pathologists.

"I got reports, hundreds of them, and figured the costs" for the pathologists.

One day as her supervisor was checking her reports, she told him she was ready for a change. She said she thought she would like to work in pathology rather than accounting.

And she made him a promise: "If I don't like it, I will quit." She didn't quit.

There was a lot of paper involved in those early days, and she handled plenty of it in pathology reports. Van Vorous was working in the original location, the old General Hospital, and was on an upper floor. The pathologist with whom she worked went out one day, and she opened a window to get some air. She got a lot of air, and it blew the reports out the window.

"I crawled out on the roof, and he came back" while she was out there. He simply laughed as she retrieved all the papers.

As the company began to spread out more with new acquisitions, Van Vorous said Dr. Jim Powell decided that someone was needed to supervise all the affiliated pathologists. He asked her to handle that assignment, which took her all across the United States. She recalls, "I worked with a lot of very smart people."

Pathologists she dealt with were medical doctors who, for example, read slides for biopsies for Pap smears, for fluid drained off a knee—and some were called to do autopsies. The first full-time pathologist with the company was Dr. George Rinker, now deceased, and she enjoyed her association with him. "He was a great teacher, and I was a good listener."

She looks back on her career with great pride.

"I started at minimum wage. People believed in me, and I retired as vice president of an S&P 500 company."

Van Vorous also developed great respect for Dr. Jim Powell. "He had a unique ability to surround himself with good people, and he gave opportunities to them" to advance and grow with the company. He was always supportive of the community and projects that would help the community. If you were working on such a project, she said, he would give you time off and you would be paid and would not have to make up the time.

"He believed in his employees and he rewarded loyalty. It broke my heart when he left," she said.

Van Vorous recalls one occasion in which she had to fire a pathologist. She flew out to the Midwest and met with him, not knowing how he would react. However, all went well as he told her, "I am glad it was you [who came to fire him]. I know I will be leaving with some dignity."

Ernie Knesel's Role

Ernie Knesel continued to be a vital part of the operations of Biomedical Laboratories. Jim Powell was serving in the military when Biomedical Laboratories was opened in 1969, and someone else had to actually organize the laboratory and provide the leadership necessary to get things going. Ernie Knesel filled that role.

While Jim Powell was away in the military, Ed and John were at Carolina Biological Supply Company (CBSC) across town. Ernie was supervisor of the labs, and he became the first vice president who was not a member of the Powell family. Ed was in on the startup and was a board member for a number of years, but was not in management. John would remain at CBSC, but worked part-time in the lab management.

"We grew from there," Knesel said. "We started in one room, then two, then one floor, then the whole building. Then we expanded to York Court."

Knesel became one of the top executives in the company as it was growing. He became head of innovation and led the development of a number of projects with international medical device companies such as Olympus in Japan. One of his projects was to develop a thin-layer system to replace and improve the fifty-year-old Pap smear for the detection of cervical cancer. That effort was formed as a separate company, Auto Cyte, which later became Tripath.

Years later, Knesel became a successful entrepreneur in his own right. He formed Select Laboratories in Greensboro, North Carolina. He started from scratch and grew to the point that he acquired a Raleigh, North Carolina, laboratory to add to his operations.

His wife, Lynn, and son, Brad, were a part of the growth of that company, and then he had a very successful exit from the operations several years ago. Since then he has founded several additional companies in the laboratory field. He and Brad continue to grow those operations.

It was not long before Biomedical Laboratories outgrew the facilities at the old hospital site. As a result, the company began construction on a seventy-thousand-square-foot building in December 1976. It was built on the opposite side of Burlington from the original site on Powell family land across the railroad tracks from Carolina Biological. It became known as the York Court facility.

The twenty acres later became forty acres after more land was acquired, and the site now is home to the largest commercial laboratory in the country under one roof. Cost of the building was $2 million, with an additional $2 million spent on new laboratory equipment.

Laboratory space was designed to be unlike anything in a traditional or a commercial laboratory at the time. It had to house an electronic, automated, and computerized laboratory that was totally different from the traditional hospital lab with multiple rows of lab benches. A large computer room was central to the facility, housing the Unisys computer that controlled and communicated lab testing from all over the Southeast in one large machine. This concept of information system centralization was new to the laboratory world, and it was spearheaded by Biomedical Laboratories.

The machine had to receive lab data, do quality control, and communicate the results back to the physician in less than twenty-four hours.

This new location housed 680 employees as well as the pathologists—the laboratory medical doctors and PhDs who oversaw the work of the lab.

The new facility was dedicated in August 1978, with US congressman Richardson Preyer in attendance.

Air Transportation for Specimens

As time passed, Biomedical Laboratories began to expand beyond Burlington and North Carolina. Cities such as Atlanta; Roanoke, Virginia; Charlotte; and Columbia, South Carolina, became a part of the operations, and while growth was good, it created a problem. The distances to those locations and others prohibited delivering twenty-four-hour service to hospitals and physicians by highway couriers.

The problem was quickly solved, however, with the airplane.

Biomedical Laboratories purchased a Cessna 210 and sent it on nightly trips to those distant locations. The plane brought specimens to the Burlington laboratory late at night or early in the morning. The specimens would be analyzed and results were immediately telecommunicated back to the healthcare provider for patient treatment.

Officials at Biomedical realized that Burlington is an ideal location for a centralized laboratory due to its easy access to all points in North Carolina and the Southeast. Two interstate highways, I-85 and I-40, run through Alamance County, and they

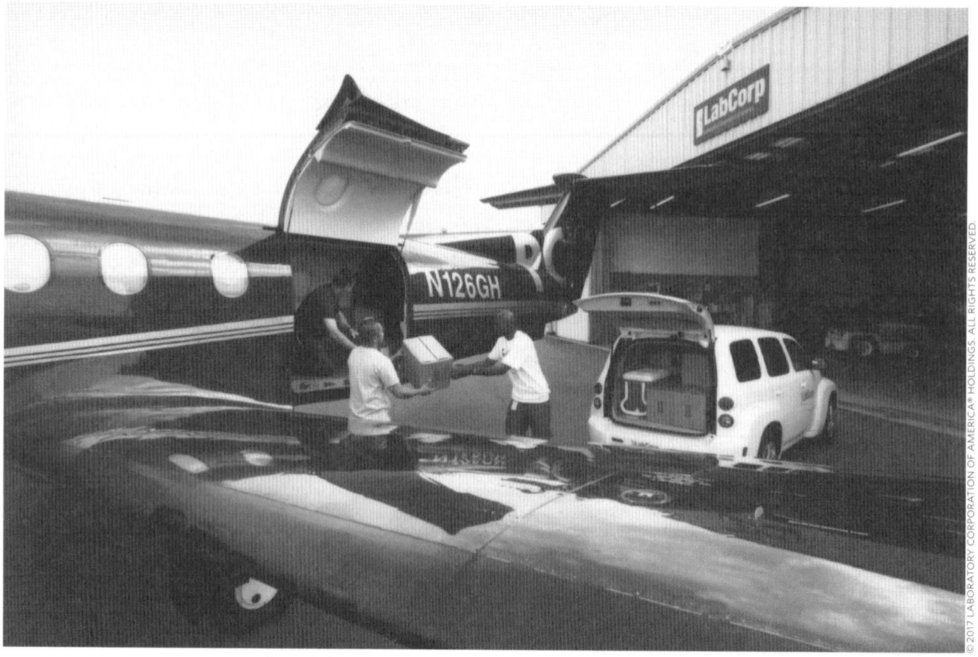

A fleet of planes has been vital part of company's operations

facilitate van delivery of specimens. Burlington is situated between Raleigh-Durham Airport and Piedmont Triad Airport in Greensboro. Charlotte's airport is but two hours away.

Even more important is the presence of Burlington's own airport. Over the years it has grown into a major base of operations for business aircraft. There is a long, modern runway and a navigational system to allow fewer weather delays, earlier delivery, and safe flying for the company's pilots. Biomedical Laboratories built the first large hangar at the airport, making it possible to have several planes and to have a full-time staff of mechanics to service the planes and keep them in the air.

As deliveries increased, it was necessary to add more planes. By the time LabCorp was formed in 1995, there was a Piper Pa-23 Aztec, two Cessna Navahos, a Beechcraft King Air, and a Cessna jet. Those planes are used every night for specimen transport, and the King Air and the Cessna jet are available during daylight hours for executive use.

Early in its history, Biomedical Laboratories found a shortage of trained laboratory assistants, so the company established a training program at Elon College. There were just not enough trained laboratory technicians in central North Carolina in the early 1970s. Traditional programs in hospitals trained technicians in the customary manual lab methods. That education was not what was needed by the new company. Knowledge of automation, electronics, and computers was essential, so laboratory training was begun at Elon College in 1974. In addition to that training course, Biomedical Laboratories began an additional training course at Elon College for cytotechnologists in the fall of 1980.

The medical technologist training course begun at Elon was a two-year course with graduates receiving an associate of science degree. The course ran successfully for a number of years, but soon it was realized that this type of training was more appropriate at Alamance Community College (ACC). The program was transferred there, and it continues to this day to provide graduates for work at LabCorp as well as at local hospitals in Alamance County and at other locations in North Carolina and other states.

The biotechnology course at ACC is currently one of the oldest in the nation. Ron Sturgill, then a senior vice president with Roche Biomed, was instrumental in its development. He served on the board of trustees there for fourteen years. The college has recently completed a lengthy and comprehensive study to determine what it would designate as its "Center of Excellence." ACC ultimately chose the biotechnology department to be designated as such.

Many of the employees in Burlington were graduates of the local public schools, and many of them had the benefit of continuing their education at ACC. The company participated in the local education program at all levels, and special attention was given to ACC. The company donated much of the equipment needed to start the programs. It was a good investment, as many of the students who studied in that ACC program later worked for Roche Biomedical Laboratories, which would follow Biomedical Laboratories.

Building on this success at ACC for technologist training, another program was started in biotechnology. That was followed by an electronics course designed for maintenance and repair of medical equipment and instruments.

Pearlie Jeffers, assistant vice president of Roche Biomedical Laboratories' electronics department, chaired an advisory committee for the biomedical equipment technology program. Students were able to learn in that program how to repair and maintain the highly sophisticated equipment used in medical laboratories, hospitals, and industrial testing laboratories. That was one of the very first such programs in the entire United States.

Mike Moore was assistant vice president of facilities engineering at Roche Biomedical in the early 1990s, and he was a graduate of ACC with an associate degree in business administration. He served on ACC's advisory committees for industrial management technology and biomedical equipment technology.

The Powell Building at ACC is now the home for allied health and biotechnology at ACC. A number of years ago, the Powell family recognized the importance of biotechnology in the community. As a result it established The Thomas E. Powell Jr. Endowment to support those activities, and that support continues to this day. In recognition of the importance of biotechnology training for the community, there are plans to more than double the space of the Powell building.

ACC is actively building its capabilties in additional technologies. An entirely new technology center is to be constructed soon, which will include mechatronics—the combining of mechanical, electrical, and computer engineering. Biotechnology is increasingly dependent on mechanotronics nanotechnology. There are a number of mechatronics programs in North Carolina, including locations in Guilford County as well as at North Carolina State University and UNC-Asheville.

CHAPTER FOUR

Good Years for Biomedical Laboratories

THE FIRST TEN YEARS HAD BEEN GOOD years for Biomedical Laboratories. The company was making an annual profit of $2 million on revenues of $18 million. That looked good on paper, but when company officials looked at the clinical laboratory market nationwide, they realized they could not sit still. The market was heating up, and certain other laboratories were growing by acquisition, just as Biomedical Laboratories was.

Biomedical Laboratories officials saw a number of other opportunities for growth through additional acquisitions—acquisitions that would help them grow, not only as a presence in the southeastern United States, but also on the national level.

Such expansion was going to require more capital, and the company's bank line was being fully utilized. The only other source of income for expansion, other than from angel investors, was from the public markets. The needed funds for expansion could be obtained by an initial public offering (IPO) as well as additional offerings as a public company if needed in the future.

There was also a desire to further extend stock ownership to company employees. Biomedical already had a profit sharing plan dating from 1974, but officials wanted to go a step further and institute an employee stock ownership plan, or ESOP.

This would be accomplished by a publicly marketed stock with a defined value that could be obtained daily in the public financial markets. The ESOP would allow employees to have a "piece of the rock" themselves.

Biomedical also believed in extending stock ownership well down into the management ranks instead of just at the top. Equity, then as today, was highly valued by the most capable managers, and this move would allow the laboratory to recruit and retain top employees, managers, and executives. This attitude has resulted in scores of managers in the company becoming independently well off. The ESOP was established on October 9, 1978, for all full-time employees. An IPO also allowed liquidity for shareholders.

The newly named Biomedical Reference Laboratories (BRL) had three outside directors during the approximately three years it was a public company. Dr. Jim Powell said the company was fortunate to have their services during that time: Ash Pipkin, Dr. Tom Keller, and Dr. Robert Sing.

Pipkin was a graduate of UNC–Chapel Hill and then received an MBA from Harvard and a law degree from Duke University. He not only brought a financial and legal background to the board, he also brought experience in information systems gained during work with Exxon in New York prior to entering the legal profession in Raleigh. Dr. Powell said, "His assistance in building the national information systems for finance and the laboratory system was invaluable."

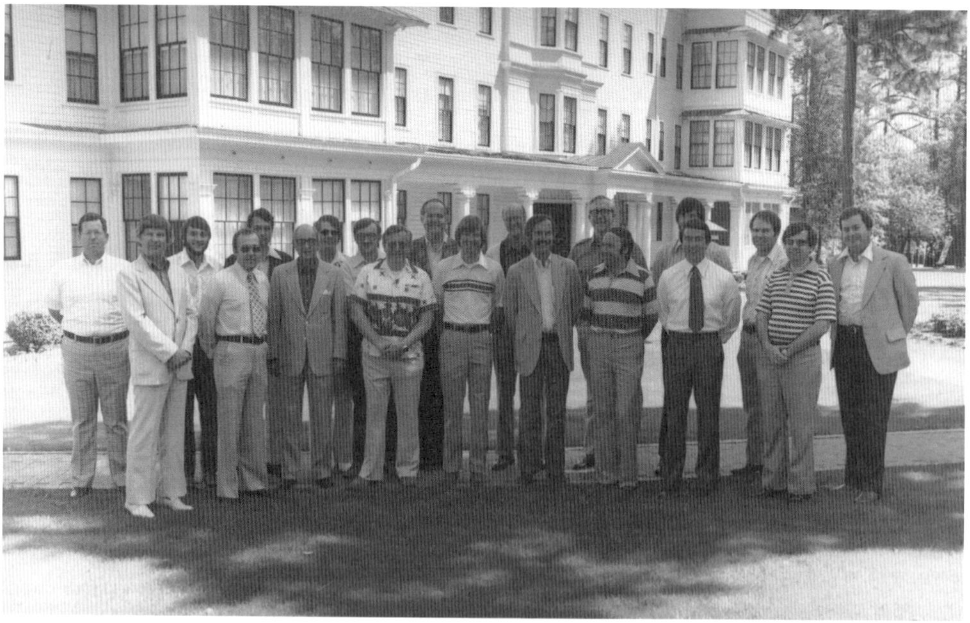

Third annual BRL sales meeting at Pinehurst NC—left to right front row: Robbie Roberson, David Weavil, Hinton Rountree, Ernie Knesel, Bill Roberts, Dr. Jim Powell, Dr. Boris Datnow, Haywood Cochrane, Bill Winstead, Wayne Kempff. Second row: Elmer Walker, Jim Folks, Paul Hoffner, Bill Irwin, Claude Armstrong, Dr. Ed Powell, Jim Spence, John Powell, Bill Kirkpatrick and Jim Creech

Dr. Keller had extensive financial experience as a CPA. He was also the founding dean of the Fuqua School of Business at Duke University.

Dr. Robert Sing was a pathologist who had founded Diagnostics Laboratories, a clinical laboratory in Charlotte. Dr. Sing had extensive experience in many of the specialty assays performed in the laboratory. His company had become a part of BRL a few years earlier.

In the early 1970s, Haywood Cochrane was with Wachovia Bank and Trust in the North Carolina Piedmont, responsible for credit accounts in the bank's northern region. He had heard of Biomedical Laboratories and was acquainted with the elder Dr. Thomas Powell. Later he worked with the Powell brothers on several projects.

"I made the loan for the first expansion on Rainey Street," and "I made the loan for the York Court" facility as well.

He found himself meeting with the brothers on a number of occasions, as they sought his advice on financial matters. Finally, one day after hearing his advice on an issue, there came a question: "How would you like to join us as chief financial officer?" He was living in Greensboro at the time and had a family, and he said he could use the additional money that the move offered. He took the job. Cochrane would be one of several people who would be introduced to Biomedical Laboratories while working for another company doing business with the lab. On April 1, 1977, he began working with Biomedical Laboratories, and with Jim Powell in particular. He got there just in time to help guide the movement to a publicly held company.

"We restructured Biomed and cleaned it up" financially, he said.

Then in 1982 Cochrane and Jim Powell negotiated the sale of Biomedical Reference Labs—the name of the company after going public—to Hoffmann-La Roche, which led to Roche Biomedical Laboratories (RBL).

"Jim Powell did an artful job of merging the cultures" represented in the two companies that came together, Cochrane said, "and that was no small job."

Action leading to this merger actually started when Biomedical's board of directors made the decision in the fall of 1978 to begin exploring avenues for the IPO. E. F. Hutton was selected for discussions regarding their being the lead underwriter.

A presentation was made to Biomedical Labs executives in New York City on January

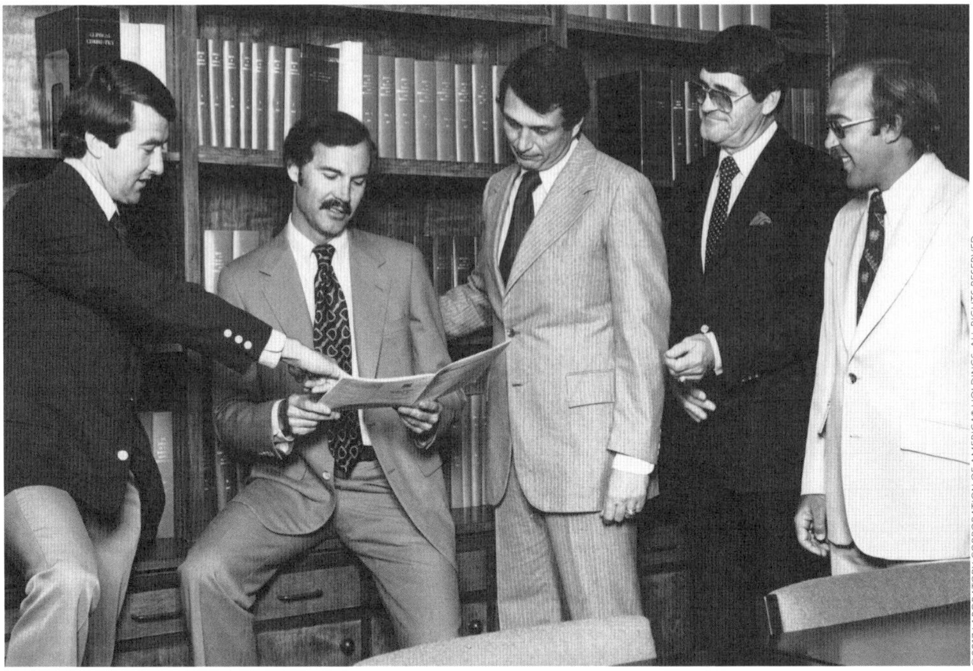

A group of early BRL managers, left to right, Haywood Cochrane, Dr. Jim Powell, Paul Hoffner, Fred Miller, Dave Weavil

4, 1979, to allow both sides to determine if the arrangement was to be a good fit. On March 6 that same year, an agreement was reached for Hutton to be the lead underwriter and for Wheat First Securities of Richmond, Virginia, to be the secondary underwriter. Wheat First Securities was chosen because of its strong regional presence in the Southeast, where primary investor interest was expected. Biomedical Laboratories thus benefitted from both national and regional underwriting, which was unusual at the time.

Underwriters and executives of Biomedical Laboratories immediately entered into due diligence for the IPO. There was a problem, however. It was discovered that the name "Biomedical Laboratories" was already in use by another laboratory in the United States. Therefore, the company had to come up with a new and unique name.

The easiest and most reasonable change seemed to be to simply insert "Reference" into the name. Thus was born Biomedical Reference Laboratories (BRL).

After an intense due diligence process, including a number of all-night sessions among all those concerned, the "red herring" or preliminary prospectus was printed on March 30, 1979, with all information except the pricing.

A few days later, after still more study and consideration, the final prospectus was printed effective May 4, 1979, with a public offering price of $13.50 per share. A total of 530,000 shares sold on the NASDAQ stock exchange, and total funds raised were slightly over $7 million. At the time of the IPO and the changing of the name, the company had offices in every southeastern state and actual laboratories in many of those states.

The IPO proved to be a good move, as growth continued rapidly. In January 1981, Biomedical Reference Laboratories had become one of the four largest commercial clinical laboratories in the United States.

Diagnostic Clinical Laboratories (DCL) in Charlotte was acquired from Dr. Robert Sing as the 1980s began. DCL had 165 employees in five states and sales of more than $5 million in fiscal 1980.

Several DCL employees became mainstays in the management ranks of Biomedical Reference Labs and its successor companies. Ron Sturgill and Jim Kilgore were two of those who joined the company from DCL. Sturgill had moved from his previous supply company work to DCL, where he was general manager. His jobs were to run the operation and expand it as well. He was made a vice president.

"We were in direct competition with the Burlington group," he said.

It was in 1986, several years after Biomedical Laboratories had become Roche Biomedical, that Sturgill was asked to move to New Jersey, where he was head of the company's North Central Division. He became a senior vice president at that time.

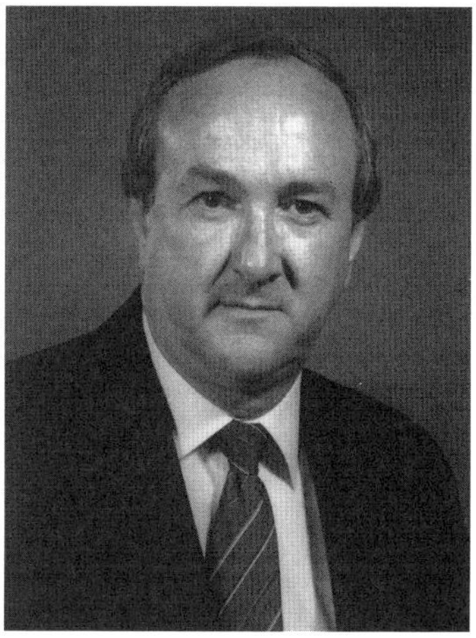

Ron Sturgill

His stay there was short, though, as he was soon called back to Burlington to head human resources, information systems, and marketing with the position of executive vice president.

When LabCorp became a reality, Sturgill continued with human resources and also headed operations in the Southeast Division. He remained as head of that division until his retirement in November 2001.

"It was quite a ride," he remembered with much pride.

As Sturgill looked back on his years with the company, he pointed to one particular event that he considered the most significant in his time there. It was the addition of the Roche name to the operations.

When the merger created Roche Biomedical Laboratories, the entire industry took note. That made the company a real player in the laboratory industry, he said. "It was phenomenal what the Roche name meant" in the industry.

In its early years, Biomedical Reference Labs had made a number of acquisitions, Sturgill explained, "and they got the attention of Roche."

At that time, he said, Roche management had decided to either "really get in or get out of the laboratory testing business." They needed skilled and experienced management, and that's when they looked seriously at Burlington.

"The management team [in Burlington] was the key to the move," Sturgill said.

He gave an example of how important the Roche name was. While he was in New Jersey, he said that if he required the attention of a doctor, he was never charged when they learned he was working for Roche.

"We gained a big market share because of that name," he added.

In 1982, through rapid internal growth and acquisitions, the client base for BRL had grown to more than ten thousand physicians.

Not only was there growth in size of the operation but in the types of testing as well.

The company became a leader in paternity testing in the early 1980s. It had been suggested in earlier years that maternity was a matter of fact and paternity was a matter of opinion. But with testing using advanced genetic techniques, opinion was replaced by fact, and the company played a major role in that process in ensuing years.

Often individuals in the paternity testing division were called upon to testify in paternity court cases to explain this new science and what it could and could not prove.

It was a paternity case in 1982 that brought national attention to the company. There was a court case in Pine Bluff, Arkansas, contesting child support involving a set of twins. When the case went to court, the defendant claimed he was not the father of the twins and he agreed to laboratory tests to prove his argument. By that time Biomedical Reference Laboratories had become Roche Biomedical Laboratories.

The human leukocyte antigen test was done in Burlington, and the report brought a surprise. It was found that there was a 99.13 percent chance that the defendant was the father of one of the twins, and there was a zero chance that he was the father of the second one.

The test involved samples of blood of the mother, the child, and the alleged father. While it could not prove paternity, the test could rule out fatherhood or give the likelihood of parentage.

A doctor testified in the trial and said it was possible for the second child to have been conceived by a second father within sixty days of the first and for the babies to be born as fraternal twins.

By 1980 Biomedical Reference Laboratories was gaining recognition in the national business community as one of the little-known companies "that flourish in specialized markets."

In 1980, the idea of merger and consolidation of smaller labs was growing in popularity, and in fact, Biomedical Reference Laboratories was looking for possible activity in that area. The idea was floated in early 1980 to merge with German pharmaceutical company Boehringer Ingelheim, which operated BioScientia Laboratory. Officials from BRL went to Germany to make an in-depth study of the company as a potential merger partner.

In a report on the visit, Ernie Knesel and Jim Geyer noted that "our visit to BioScientia was very interesting, and although we found their laboratory to be behind Biomedical in most respects, especially automation, we did gain valuable information in regard to some specific ways they handle their specimens and procedures." They also saw European countries as a good source for "very expensive and unobtainable chemicals" as well as certain "expensive and valuable antibodies." It was a most favorable report, and the deal moved to a proposed closing in New York City, but the merger fell through at that point.

By early 1982, Biomedical Reference Laboratories was extremely busy in the area of acquisitions. In a period of just fifteen months, the company had added seven other laboratories, and major consolidations were taking place in the industry across the nation. In that business climate, Biomedical Reference Laboratories agreed to become a part of the third major consolidation in the industry in the six months leading to March 1982.

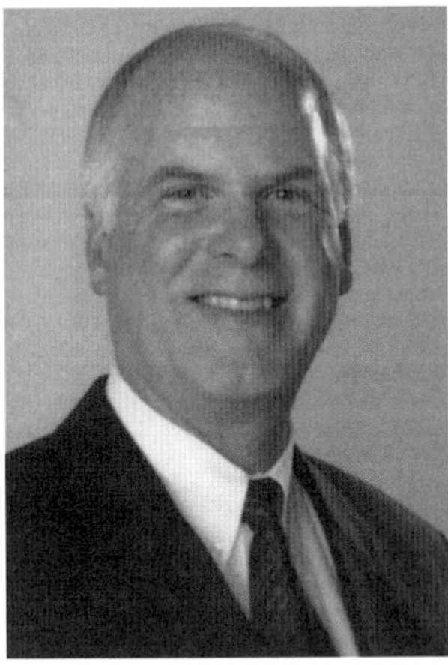

Wes Elingburg

As one more among many examples, Wes Elingburg was with another company doing work that put him in contact with Biomedical Laboratories, leading to his employment with Biomed.

Elingburg had graduated from Western Carolina University in accounting in 1978 and was employed with Peat Marwick Mitchell in Greensboro. Biomedical was an audit client for that firm, and Elingburg was on the audit team. He did that for a couple of years and then was asked to become a part of Biomedical Laboratories. David Weavil had made that same move a few years earlier. In fact, Weavil hired him at Biomedical.

Elingburg was director of financial reporting, arriving just in time to be part of the move to a publicly traded company. Then in 1982 he had a role in the purchase of the company by Hoffmann–La Roche.

Elingburg remembers a Saturday in the fall of 1982 when he was at home watching football, dressed in a football jersey and jeans. He received a call from Jim Powell telling him there was urgent business at the Burlington office and Elingburg needed to be there.

"I got there, and there were Roche people all over, wearing suits," but he got into the action and helped the company become Roche Biomedical Laboratories. He became senior vice president of finance for that new company. That move brought a different atmosphere to the company, he said. "The whole world changed."

The Biomedical operation had more of a family feeling, and "it was incredibly well run." Elingburg said Roche was also a good company, and he made many friends in both New Jersey and in Basel, Switzerland, where Roche was headquartered.

"They let us run the company," he said, and "were great to work with."

CHAPTER FIVE

A New Company Is Born

ON MARCH 22, 1982, IT WAS ANNOUNCED that Biomedical Reference Laboratories would become a part of Hoffmann–La Roche Inc.

Irwin Lerner, president of Hoffmann–La Roche in the United States, and Dr. James Powell, president of BRL, announced the agreement. No changes in management of BRL were anticipated, and Lerner stated that he looked forward to continued success at the North Carolina laboratory operation under Dr. Powell's leadership.

At the time of the announcement, it was reported that a definitive agreement had been reached with holders of approximately 31 percent of BRL's stock, and that Hoffman-La Roche would pay them $28 per share for 5.8 million shares, or $163.5 million.

When Biomedical had gone public in 1979, it showed a profit of 20 percent, largest of any lab in the country, according to Ernie Knesel, vice president of lab operations at the time. He said Roche officials had seen that and took great interest, as their clinical laboratory company had not shown a profit from 1969 through 1982. Knesel explained that the Swiss ownership of Roche viewed that situation and said "make it profitable or get rid of it," so Lerner decided to buy Biomedical in an effort to make things profitable.

Knesel gave Irwin Lerner much credit for the success of the move. Dr. Jim Powell also praised Lerner for his leadership in making the BRL–Hoffman–La Roche deal a reality.

Lerner's agreement to purchase Biomedical came after a thorough analysis of the industry. Thomas Mac Mahon was an analyst with Roche at the time, and he was told

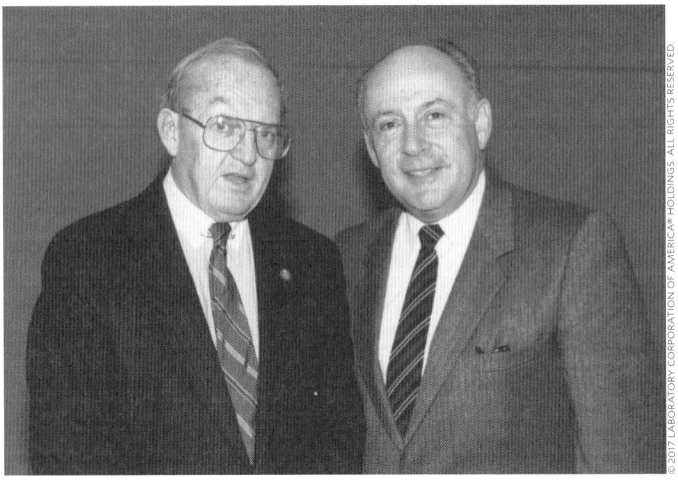

Irwin Lerner of Roche with Congressman Howard Coble at a company event

to look around and see what other businesses were out there dealing in diagnostic products. He was to do analyses of those companies, and "that's when I found Biomedical," Mac Mahon said. He would later become president, CEO, and board chair of LabCorp soon after it formed in the 1990s.

By 1982 the national media recognized that big corporations were getting into the clinical laboratory business. The industry was growing rapidly, and there were many mom-and-pop operations being acquired and merged into much larger companies. Bigger companies had technology and resources that smaller companies found hard to match.

One lab president said, "Once you could get into this business for about $200,000. Now one machine costs $300,000."

It indeed was a time for mergers, and experts agreed that the Biomedical Reference Laboratories and Hoffmann–La Roche move was a good one. A North Carolina security analyst said at the time that Hoffmann–La Roche was "buying the best company in the industry, from a management standpoint, an operating standpoint, and a statistical standpoint." He said the management team was the best in the industry.

Hoffmann–La Roche is an international company dealing in pharmaceuticals and diagnostics. It has headquarters in Basel, Switzerland. The company was founded in 1896 by Fritz Hoffmann–La Roche and in 2014 had 88,509 employees with revenue of $48 billion.

At the time of the union with Hoffmann–La Roche, Biomedical Reference Laboratories was operating in twenty-two states, most of them in the South. There were 1,700 employees at seventy-two branches, twenty-three immediate analysis labs, and seven more advanced regional labs. In the previous year the company had tested 4.8 million specimens, such as blood and body tissue, for 15,500 doctors, hospitals, and clinics.

Hoffmann–La Roche had entered the clinical laboratory business in 1969 when it purchased Kings County Research Laboratories (KCRL) in Brooklyn, New York, forming Roche Clinical Laboratories (RCL). That laboratory in Brooklyn had been operated by a renowned endocrinologist and pioneer in fertility treatments, Herbert S. Kuppermann, MD, PhD.

Bernadette (Bunny) Ventura-Warfell remembered Dr. Kuppermann well. She was his medical assistant at one time, and she was a part of the transition of Kings County Research Laboratories into Roche Clinical Laboratory, then to Roche Biomedical, and eventually into LabCorp.

Dr. Kuppermann's lab first was in Brooklyn, then West Caldwell, New Jersey. "It was a beginning," Ventura-Warfell said. They had all the various departments they needed, and then suddenly came the merger with RCL.

"KCRL closed the doors one night, and the next day employees found they had moved to Raritan [New Jersey]," she said. She stayed in hematology for several years and then became a manager.

"We grew rapidly," she said, especially in patient services.

Later Ventura-Warfell became involved in recruitment and then was an instructor in many lab disciplines. She lived in New Jersey, but her work took her from Virginia to the Canadian border. She ended her career as a coding instructor. Every procedure in the testing process has to be coded, she said—a vital step in the process. She retired in 2005 after thirty-five years with the company.

When the Roche purchase was made, Dick Murphy became a familiar face to those in Burlington. He was an executive vice president at Roche in the United States, and he became a member of the Roche executive committee that was responsible for diagnostics and laboratory operations in the United States.

Jim Powell said, "Dick was a thoroughly likeable individual who was well received by the management at RBL. He worked well with all the executives in the newly formed company." Powell said he was quite comfortable with Murphy and had no problem with any of his direct reports, nor did he have a problem if Murphy had conversations in which he was not a part. Powell explained, "There was a feeling of collegiality that is rare in corporate America today."

The CBL Purchase

Just a few months after Roche purchased RBL in 1982, it was announced that Roche had also purchased Consolidated Biomedical Laboratories Inc. (CBL) in Columbus, Ohio. Ernie Knesel said that after the successful purchase of Biomedical, the Swiss owners said, "'Go buy something else.' They had bought us and our success."

Soon after announcement of the Consolidated purchase, Biomedical Reference Laboratories, Consolidated Biomedical Laboratories, and Roche Clinical Laboratories joined to become Roche Biomedical Laboratories, with reference testing facilities in Burlington, North Carolina; Columbus, Ohio; and Raritan, New Jersey. Dr. James B. Powell was named president and CEO of Roche Biomedical.

The purchase of Consolidated was a move of major significance for BRL. Knesel said that Consolidated was spread all across the country, and the purchase of that company made Roche Biomedical a national operation for the first time. Several others who were a part of the company at that time expressed the same feeling, noting it to be a major step in the growth of Roche Biomedical Laboratories.

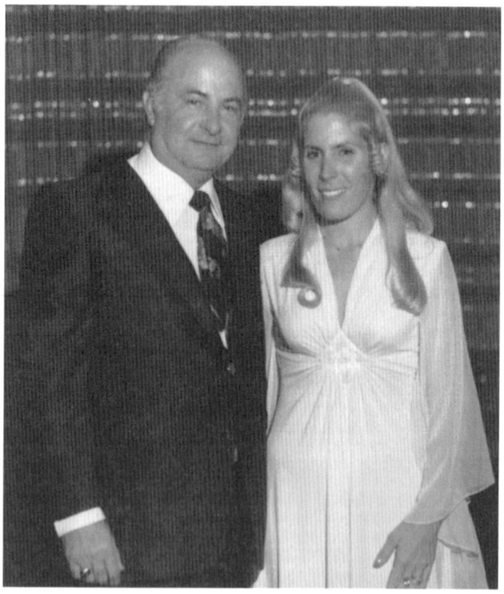

Linda Smith with Jack Walsh, vice president, sales, Consolidated Biomedical Laboratories at 1978 annual meeting

At the time of the purchase of Consolidated, Linda Smith had been with that laboratory since 1975. She said it had started in the early 1970s as a veterinary laboratory and soon became a wholly owned subsidiary of Rohm and Haas. That company also owned Micro Medic Systems, offering RIA Lab instrumentation.

Smith said CBL initially pursued the local physician community as clients and spread out to cover most of Ohio. She was hired as a district manager in

Miami, Florida, in 1975 to open that state's market. Her job included promoting and offering esoteric testing to hospitals, researchers, and smaller private labs. She was also responsible for setting up logistics to pick up the specimens from clients and ensure that they were transported to the Columbus laboratory "according to specimen integrity mandates."

"Our success in doing this paved a way for CBL to be very competitive with all other esoteric labs," she said.

This also led to collaboration with researchers in Florida medical schools for pharmaceutical studies. The result was the launch of a clinical trial program in Florida that eventually was promoted throughout CBL.

CBL was growing in the late 1970s, acquiring laboratories in Wichita, Virginia, Denver, and Sacramento.

"Each of these laboratory acquisitions not only brought market share and improved logistics" but also added laboratories "nationally known for expertise in many areas of testing," Smith said.

In 1980 Smith moved to Columbus to become a regional field manager for the East Coast as well as for Alabama, Louisiana, Kentucky, Tennessee, Michigan, Indiana, and Ohio. Her mission was the same as in Florida: "secure esoteric testing and set up logistics to ensure specimens were in our Columbus laboratory the same day they were drawn. Our turnaround time of results was a huge advantage over Bioscience and others. Our region soon became number one in hospital reference testing, clinical trials, and serving other labs."

With the acquisition, of course, Smith became a part of Roche Biomed, and she worked in sales and management for the rest of her career. She became sales manager based in Columbus, Ohio, and was a five-time winner of the President's Achievement Award for the number-one division. Later she was appointed vice president of sales.

When LabCorp was formed, Smith became vice president of sales for the Great Lakes Division based in Columbus, Ohio. From 1996 to 1999 she was vice president of sales and new business development, where she focused on sales and lab management and developed a client service rep program. She then moved back to Florida, where for two years she served as vice president working with a hospital and new business development team before retiring in 2001.

Peter Huley was also with Consolidated at the time of the purchase. Huley actually started his career in medical technology at a smaller company that later was taken over by Consolidated. He was with Physicians Clinical Laboratory (PCL) in Richmond, Virginia, in 1975. Prior to that Huley worked in the laboratory of Presbyterian Hospital in Charlotte, North Carolina. While there he decided he would go back to school and do graduate work in medical technology. He decided on the Medical College of Virginia in Richmond, and when a friend learned of his plans, he told Huley he could get him a job at PCL. The friend told him to just show up—that he would have a job. Huley showed up, and even though no one there knew about it, they gave him the job on his friend's word. He worked nights during the week and days on Saturday and Sunday, going to school at the same time. He was a medical technician doing testing in the laboratory. He also set up the microbiology laboratory. Eventually that small lab moved into a larger location, and "it became attractive to others" at that point.

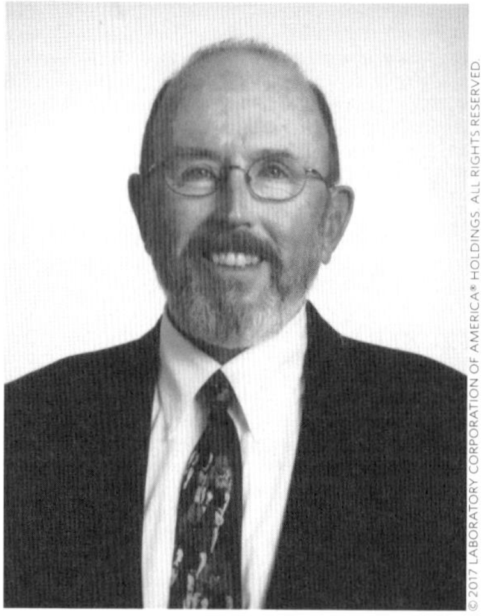

Peter Huley

Consolidated purchased PCL and was a competitor with Biomedical Reference Labs.

When Consolidated became a part of RBL, Huley was not unfamiliar with the Burlington company. While he was working at the hospital in Charlotte, Huley had received a call from BRL about a possible job offer. He and his wife visited Burlington and frankly were not impressed. The Burlington operation was then in the basement of the old hospital, and the Burlington area was rather small and quite unlike Charlotte. He kept his job in Charlotte.

He remembered then that in about 1980 he received another call to go to Burlington, but this time as part of an out-of-state inspection team. The team had been requested by Dr. Jim Powell, and Huley found himself a part of that team. On the trip to Burlington he remembered his first visit, but then the team drove up in front of the York Court operation. Much to his surprise it was "not the same place" in more ways than one. He was highly impressed with the people and the facilities.

A couple of years later Huley found himself a part of that organization when Consolidated was purchased. He went to Burlington to manage the microbiology laboratory. This time he was most impressed not only with the company but the community. He was especially impressed with the Burlington City School System, recognized as one of the top three in the state at the time.

Huley worked with Dr. Rich Hahn on a company standardization project for a while, in addition to his duties with the microbiology department as well as other areas. For several years he headed logistics and other outside operations, and he said he worked three years on plans for an addition at York Court. Things moved along, but after the formation of LabCorp, that project was brought to a sudden halt.

"We had ordered all the supplies, and we had steel lying in the yard."

The project was resumed in later years and finished in 2012. With its completion, Huley retired after thirty-eight years. At retirement he was senior vice president with responsibility for the Center for Esoteric Testing (CET), the national reference lab portion of the Burlington lab at York Court.

As the Consolidated purchase and its resulting growth were taking place, Jim Powell said, "We're becoming more and more a company that's doing sophisticated testing. We want to be on the cutting edge instead of two years late. I like new challenges. And this is a new challenge—to take this [company] forward with a lot more behind us."

Roche Biomedical offered a broad spectrum of clinical laboratory testing, including all the routine testing but also some innovative procedures not available elsewhere. More than 630 procedures covering almost every aspect of clinical laboratory testing were being performed by the company at that time. The catalog of services issued on January 1, 1984, listed every one of those procedures with the costs for each. Offered were such varied testing procedures as liver panels, viral hepatitis profiles, acid mucopolysaccharide testing, identification of cannabis sativa L. (marijuana), cholesterol testing, and hundreds of others.

Burlington was chosen for the headquarters of the new company. The city was good strategically and geographically, but it also happened to be good opportunistically as far as growth was concerned. In the early 1980s, a number of economic factors were at play in Burlington. The textile and hosiery industries were once the economic core of the community. Burlington had been the birthplace of Burlington Industries, once the largest textile producer in the world, but in the last part of the twentieth century, textiles and hosiery were in sharp decline. A large shopping mall had been built earlier just west of downtown, and that drew major department stores and variety stores from the downtown area. As their absence was felt, smaller businesses were forced to move out as well.

That left much vacant business property in the downtown area, including a large bank tower that was the city's major landmark. Built in 1929 the structure had been home to major banking companies over the years, and also in earlier years was home to doctors, dentists, attorneys, and other professionals in its nine stories.

Roche Biomedical needed space quickly. Seeing this situation as a major opportunity, Roche Biomedical took over many of those vacant buildings and moved financial and business operations into them. Smaller buildings in the downtown area were occupied in the 1980s, but the bank tower was not purchased until 1990.

The thirty-three-thousand-square-foot structure was given a total renovation and became the symbol of Roche Biomed's presence in Burlington and Alamance County. The building had been constructed as headquarters for the Atlantic Bank and Trust Co. and later was home to Security National Bank and finally NCNB.

In its renovation, the bank building was brought up to modern standards, of course, but in recognition of its historical significance, one of the floors was kept in its original 1929 configuration and decoration. The original architectural drawings for the building are displayed on that floor as well. The massive vault in the basement was also totally renovated and restored to working order.

The presence of hundreds and hundreds of Roche Biomed employees brought a renewed life to downtown Burlington, and many credited the company with saving the city. Prior to purchasing the bank building, the company had purchased the old Federal Building (post office) on Spring Street, as well as the vacant J. C. Penney building on Main Street. The former home of First Federal Savings and Loan at Davis Street and Lexington Avenue had been leased as well. The company also moved into another major piece of property in downtown, an eighty-thousand-square-foot office building that had once housed one of the major hosiery operations in the city during an era when Burlington was known as "The Hosiery Center of the South."

Thanks to the company's efforts in the downtown area, much of it is now included on the National Register of Historic Places.

Much of this spatial growth was due to new Medicare regulations in 1984 that

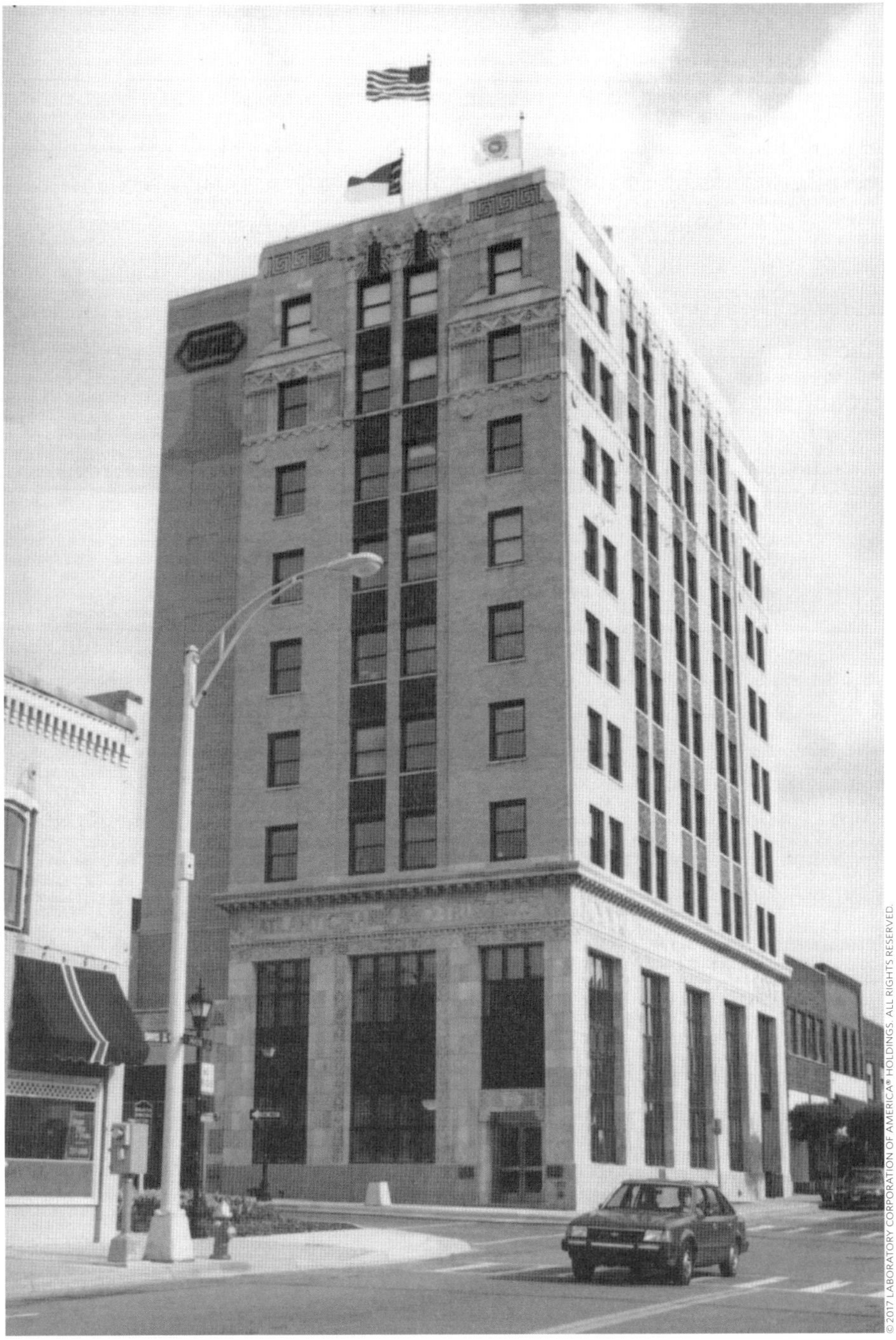

Bank tower in Burlington NC became part of RBL properties in 1990

required medical labs to provide greater billing information. This required more office space, and the vacant buildings in Burlington filled the need.

The Federal Building held a place of major significance in local history. It was constructed in 1936 as the Burlington Post Office. It was a Depression-era project of the federal government, and in the big lobby area, two large murals were painted, one at each end of the building. The murals were designed by Arthur L. Bairnsfather and were of the regionalistic style of murals painted in many public buildings across the nation in the Depression. The government sponsored the painting of the murals in an effort to make original-quality art available to the general public. One of the murals portrays a scene at the local railroad depot during the Civil War. It was the railroad that gave birth to the city in the 1850s. The mural at the other end of the building portrays the slasher room in a local textile mill, as textiles were a major industry in the town's history.

The company received a number of awards for its efforts in restoring the old buildings in downtown Burlington and putting them to a new and productive use. However, the federal government to this day retains ownership of the murals in the Federal Building.

The Circle of Excellence

RBL was growing rapidly. After the mergers of Biomedical Reference Laboratories in Burlington; Consolidated Biomedical Laboratories in Columbus, Ohio; Roche Clinical Laboratories of Raritan, New Jersey; and other expansions, RBL had become the second-largest clinical laboratory in the nation, with over nine thousand employees and nearly five hundred locations.

A major focus of the company was always the quality and abilities of its employees. RBL required technical skills for its laboratories, and beyond that, some people had to have management, sales, and marketing skills as well. It was hard to fill positions like that in a company that was growing so quickly.

Dr. Jim Powell said, "With a 24 percent growth margin in sales in the first year, the company was expanding fast, but we started to lose some of the cohesiveness we had when we were a smaller company. We began to look for someone who could get everyone to dance to the same tune—and do it quickly." To help with that problem, Roche Biomedical turned to one of the most successful small-college football coaches in the country, who happened to be right next door at Elon.

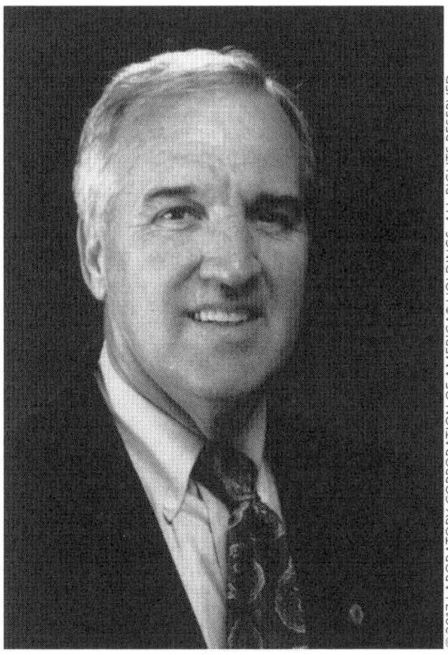

Dr. Jerry Tolley

Dr. Jerry Tolley was head football coach of Elon's NAIA team that won back-to-back national championships in 1980 and 1981. Dr. Tolley had become an assistant football coach at Elon in 1967, and ten years later he began a highly successful tenure as head coach, including two national championships. His teams won 81 percent of their games.

He retired in 1982 after his second championship and became coordinator of the college's fundraising efforts. When he started, only 15 percent of alumni were giving, but when he left in 1986 to join RBL, 48 percent were giving.

Hired in July 1986 as national coordinator of training and recruitment for RBL, Dr. Tolley developed a training program based on topics such as problem solving, leadership styles, motivation, communications, goal setting, and accounting. After Dr. Tolley joined the company, he developed a training course for "promising young managers. The goal [was] to define a corporate culture for the rapidly expanding company to assure continuity." Dr. Tolley called the training program "The Circle of Excellence." He dug into his own experiences as a student at the Fuqua School of Business Executive Education at Duke University, Vanderbilt University, and the Greensboro Center for Creative Leadership.

Dr. Jim Powell felt that Dr. Tolley's experience in game-winning strategies in football and a sophisticated understanding of business management made him just the man to create the Circle of Excellence. In a 1988 newspaper interview, Dr. Powell said, "We need to train people in sales, marketing, and technical work, and for a fast-growing company like we are, a course like this is very valuable." In a typical communication about the program to prospective attendees, the purpose of the program was stated as follows: "To provide selected LabCorp employees the opportunity to learn more about the corporation in general and to develop a wide range of managerial and leadership skills." The company wanted to groom successors for management positions, to promote career development and performance management, and to recognize and promote top performance, focusing on developing and retaining high-level staffers. Finally, a stated goal of the program was to demonstrate the company's commitment to development.

The Circle of Excellence used some unusual teaching situations to develop and grow a program that became nationally recognized. For instance, faculty included outstanding university professors who assumed the roles of such pairs as Captain Queeg and Mr. Roberts of *The Caine Mutiny* and the British and Japanese commanders in *The Bridge on the River Kwai* to help "develop improved management skills, a stronger sense of teamwork, and a company-wide perspective on the goals" of the company.

Originally the program was spread over five weekend seminars over a six-month period. Later it became an intensive weeklong seminar at Myrtle Beach, South Carolina, and there were annual reunions to review concepts and renew relationships.

Participants were chosen for leadership potential and came from all across the nation and from every educational background, from high school graduates to MBAs and PhDs. Those chosen to attend were among the top 3 percent of RBL employees by count.

As the program progressed, Dr. Tolley said, "What is surprising is the emergence of a distinctive corporate culture for the relatively young organization from the training experience."

Dr. Powell agreed, saying that one of the greatest strengths of the program was "this personal involvement in shaping the character of the company."

"Our culture is still emerging," he said. Dr. Powell noted that Roche Biomedical Laboratories represented the coming together of some sixty different entities since the company's founding nine years earlier. "We have an entrepreneurial, young culture that's distinctly our own, and Circle of Excellence participants are helping to shape it."

John Merritt, vice president of regional sales for the Mid-Atlantic Region in Burlington, said that critiquing corporate culture was one of the unique aspects of the program. He said it was personally exciting for him, as it was for so many others, to influence corporate policy and culture for the company's future.

Indeed, many others felt the same way. Participants were asked to rate the program on a scale of 1 to 5, and the average grade was 4.888. Dr. Tolley reported, "One person said this was the best training he had in eighteen years—and he graded the program lower than anyone else."

Karen McFadden, a longtime sales executive still with the company, said she learned a great deal more than she expected from Circle of Excellence. "I'm a much stronger manager now," she explained. "I've learned when to delegate and when not to. I'm also involving a lot more people in decision making."

One part of the program received particular emphasis—the mentor-protégé partnership. It was designed to foster entrepreneurial attitudes within the company. Protégés and mentors were assigned to one another. A mentor might have had several protégés, but none of the protégés worked with that mentor in daily company operations. In some cases, a protégé in one Circle of Excellence training situation might be a mentor in another.

Fred Simpson, who was senior vice president of operations in Kansas City, Missouri, at the time, said of this part of the program, "I gained a lot of information from my mentor [senior vice president Ernie Knesel at RBL in Burlington] on his decision-making techniques. He's one of the best people in the country, with the foresight to envision the results of his decisions several years down the road."

All RBL officers also participated in the program, and its success was shown in ways other than ratings. A number of those participating moved on up the ladder, and some even conducted mini-versions of the program in their own divisions.

The program attracted national attention, including from the Center for Creative Leadership, a nonprofit educational institution devoted to executive development. The center, located in Greensboro, North Carolina, featured the program in its 1990 edition of Leadership Education—A Resource Book.

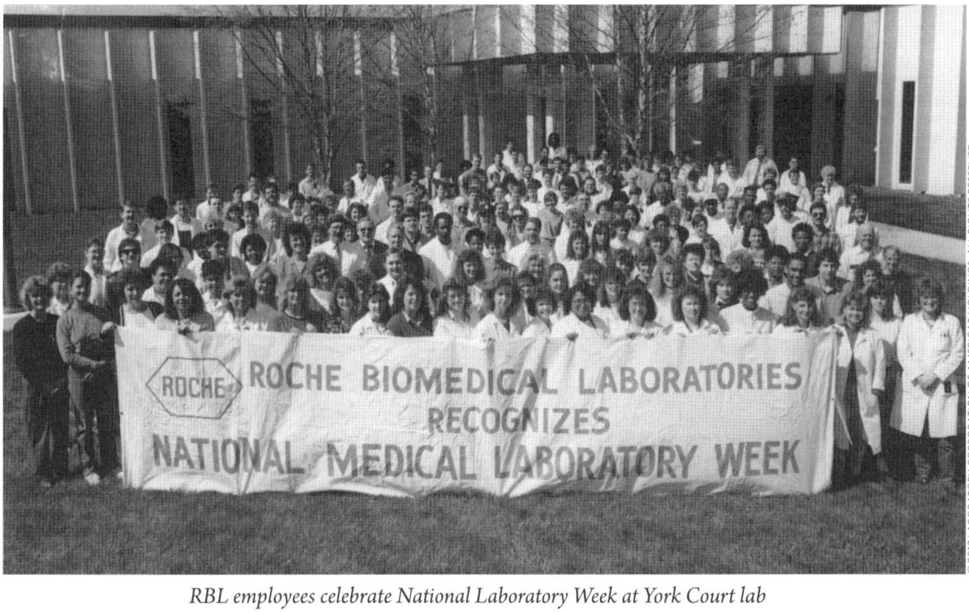

RBL employees celebrate National Laboratory Week at York Court lab

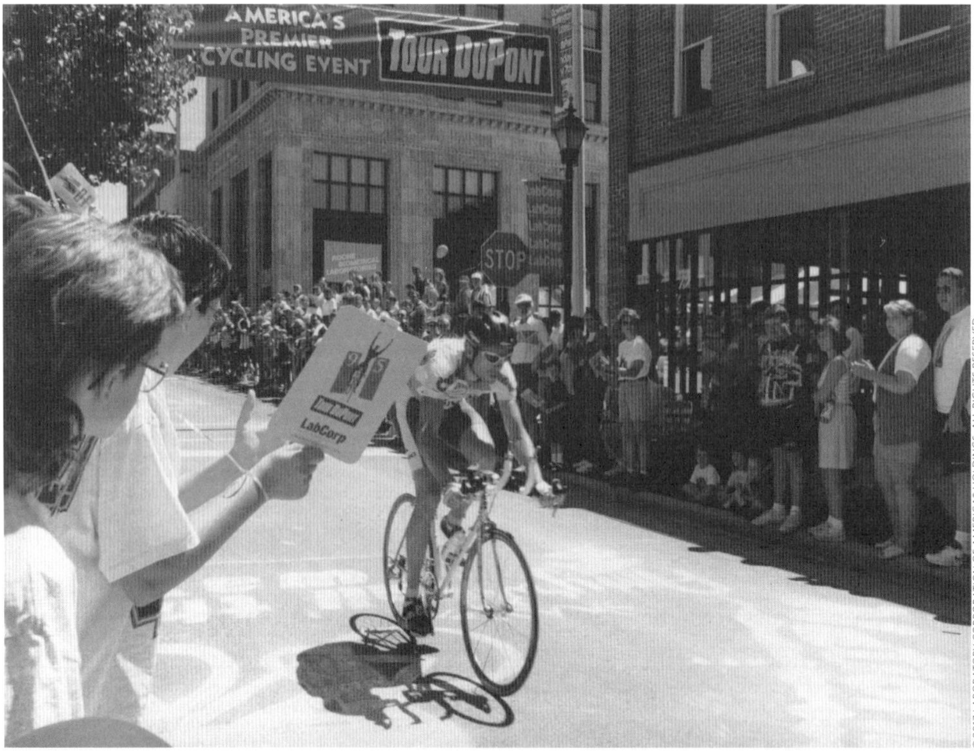

LabCorp sponsored the Tour DuPont cycling event through Burlington in 1995

Dr. Tolley also recalled that employees were encouraged to participate in community projects through volunteering or contributions of time, money, or both. The company itself, he said, was indeed active in many efforts aimed at supporting and improving the community.

Awards were given annually for teaching excellence in the local schools, and leadership workshops were given to local teachers and students. Students were sent to Washington, DC, to experience government at work, and the Roche Volunteer Program provided one thousand dollars each to local schools in the name of employees who volunteered at those schools. A long list of local agencies also benefitted from the company's contributions of time and money.

The company also supported athletic teams in various city leagues where it had operations. Karen McFadden was a member of a company softball team when she was in New Jersey. There were nine siblings in her family, and five of them worked for the company at one time or another. One of them was an outstanding softball player, so "we hired her as a ringer for our softball team. We won our league championship" the year she was hired, McFadden recalls.

The company initiated a matching-gifts program in which RBL matched all gifts made by employees to a college of their choice up to five thousand dollars. That program continues today, as do many other efforts supporting the communities in which the company has operations.

Dr. Tolley also noted the company's involvement with Alamance Community College as further indication of its commitment to the community. After his work at Roche Biomedical Laboratories, Dr. Tolley was elected mayor of Elon and he remains in that office today.

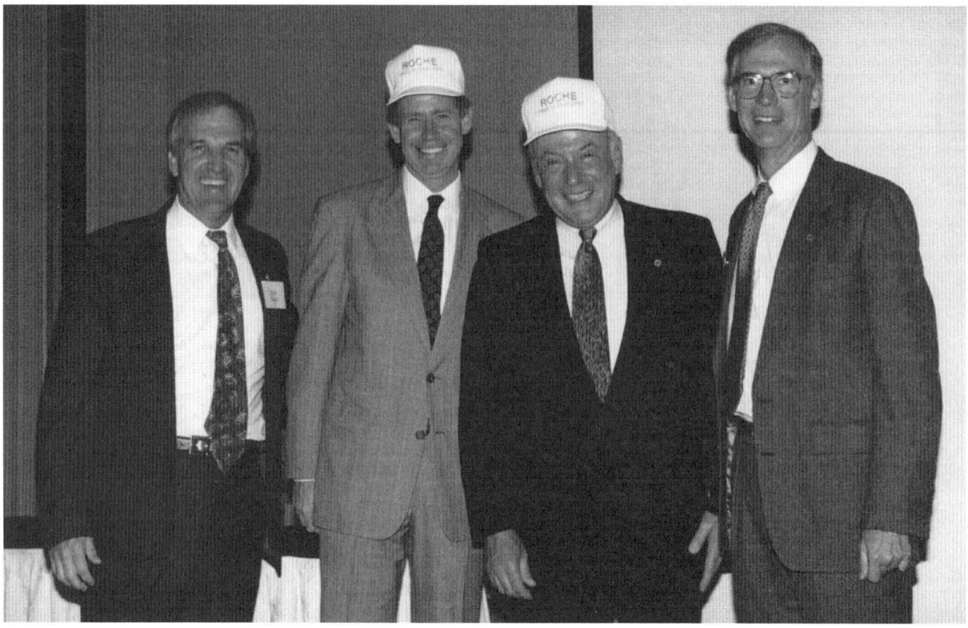

Dr. Jerry Tolley, Tom Mac Mahon, Irwin Lerner, and Dr. Jim Powell at national RBL sales award program in Florida

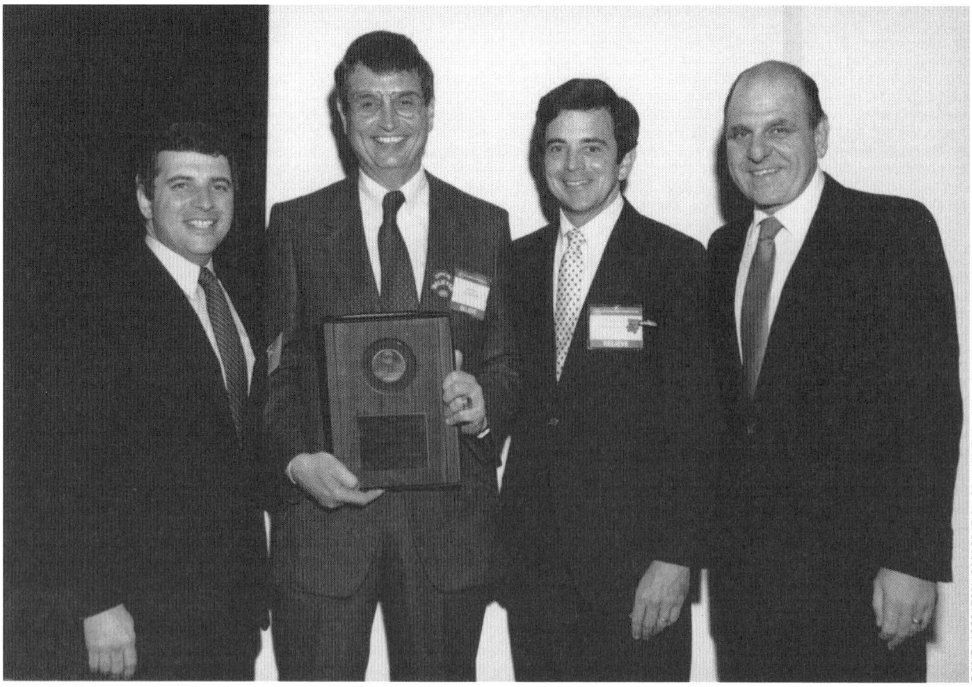

Ralph Monterosa, Paul Hoffner, John Merritt and Tom Aidala at RBL national sales meeting

CHAPTER SIX

"More Than Just a Service Lab" … and DNA

AS TIME PASSED, THE LAB GREW its testing operations, but at the same time had an eye to improve other areas of the industry. Extensive research was done in developing quicker and more sensitive diagnostic assays. Jim Powell said, "We follow the demands of the health care system, but we like to think that we are innovators also. We want to be more than just a service lab."

An area of growing concern in the 1980s was the use of drugs by employees in business and industry. Owners needed help in controlling the problem, and Roche Biomedical Laboratories stepped in to provide it. RBL joined with Pragma Bio-Tech Inc. of New Jersey to provide the workplace drug and alcohol testing that was being demanded. Under that plan, employees of Pragma would take samples from employees at their places of work and convey them to RBL. RBL would conduct sensitive chromatography / mass spectrometry tests to detect the presence of controlled substances. The results of those tests would be returned to the companies within forty-eight hours.

The drug and alcohol program was but one of the innovative moves that Roche Biomed made. Many others led to increased growth for the company, one of which was the formation of the Roche Insurance Laboratory in 1989. This operation was formed to do testing required by insurance companies to determine whether to extend coverage or to pay a claim.

The company opened yet another major facility in Research Triangle Park in August 1990. The Center for Molecular Biology would be the site for tests to detect

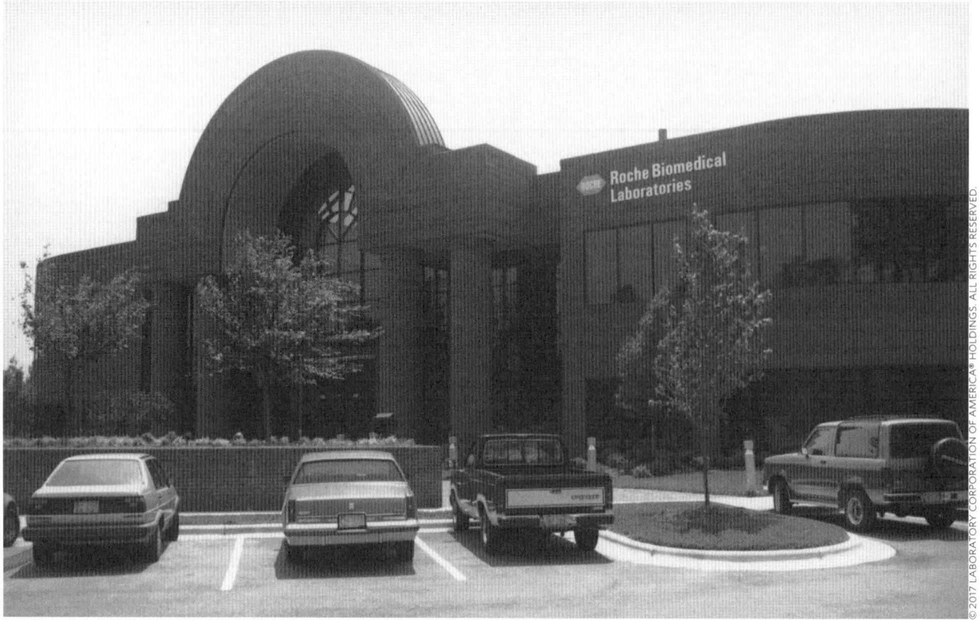

Center for Molecular Biology in Research Triangle Park, NC

substance abuse, the AIDS virus, and infectious diseases. The Polymerase Chain Reaction Laboratory was there as well, providing housing for the VAL-I.D. PCR test used to detect the presence of the human immunodeficiency virus (HIV), the virus that causes AIDS. Also included in the center was the Forensic Toxicology Laboratory, a part of the company's Substance Abuse Testing Division. This facility would become one of the most important operations in the entire company then and in years to come due to its work with PCR, the polymerase chain reaction, invented in the 1980s by Dr. Kary Mullis, a native of Lenoir, North Carolina.

Dr. Myla Lai-Goldman, a pathologist, was hired by Dr. Jim Powell to join the company on July 1, 1990, to be a part of the opening of the Center for Molecular Biology. At that time the facility did not even have a name, but its main purpose was to develop the PCR technology to its fullest. Soon the name was chosen, and Dr. Lai-Goldman became operations manager for the facility. After the laboratory opened, she became chief science officer, chief medical officer, and executive vice president of the parent company. She was also a member of the executive committee, serving until 2008 when she left to form a company in the Triangle area dealing with cancer, a company not owned by LabCorp but partially funded by it.

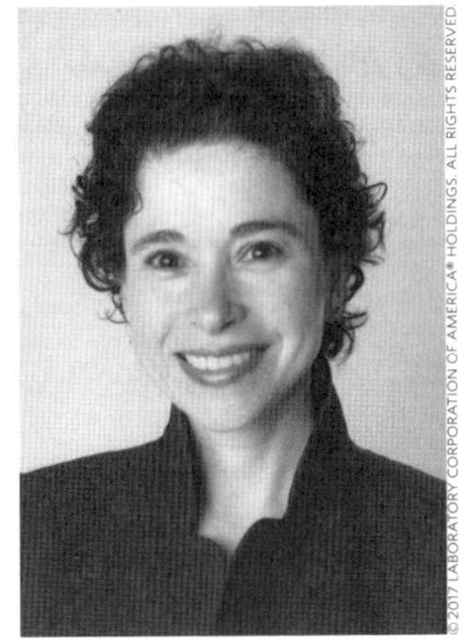

Dr. Myla Lai-Goldman

The PCR procedure developed by Dr. Mullis allowed for splitting each pair of a person's chromosomes into two. Then those strands are duplicated, and the repeating of the amplification creates millions of copies of a person's DNA. The DNA, thus amplified, can be tested in the laboratory.

By 1991 Roche Biomedical Laboratories had developed DNA technology to a point that was a breakthrough in many ways, including identification of the remains of the deceased or individuals involved in criminal investigations. This technology came at a particularly good time for Ronald Cotton, the young man mentioned at the beginning of this book who was facing a long time in prison for crimes he did not commit. DNA testing brought him his freedom and the promise of a future.

The Cotton case was not the only one to attract national and even international attention. In 2006 famed attorney-turned-bestselling-author John Grisham wrote *Innocent Man,* a book that related the story of another man who had been wrongly sentenced in Oklahoma. The man was on death row as the result of a crime committed in 1982, and a long effort was made to prove his innocence. That was finally accomplished in 1999 when evidence in the case was tested for DNA. The testing, as stated in Grisham's book, was performed by LabCorp.

DNA testing also came at a good time for the military. The United States had troops in the Middle East in Operation Desert Storm, and sometimes when military personnel were killed, identification was a problem. But DNA technology was used with outstanding results. In that process, the DNA, or the genetic fingerprint of the tissues of a body, was examined to determine identity. The laboratory was able to work with the Armed Forces Institute of Pathology to identify remains of all missing combatants in that operation. Because of this work, Desert Storm was the first military operation in which no American fighter was buried in the Tomb of the Unknown Soldier at Arlington National Cemetery. Thanks to Roche Biomedical Laboratories, there were no unknowns from that operation. Bodies of those killed were also returned to families more intact than in past conflicts.

Kary Mullis received the Nobel Prize in 1993 for his work in developing the polymerase chain reaction. He was employed at Cetus Corporation in California and had been working on the idea for some years.

Jim Powell said that the idea reportedly came to Mullis when he was driving with his girlfriend in the hill country near San Francisco one Friday night. He immediately stopped the car, got out, put a piece of paper on the hood of the car, and sketched out how the procedure would work. He took his sketch to Cetus on Monday and tried to convince his coworkers of the procedure's merits. They did not believe him, but they allowed him to use laboratory space for his work, and Mullis subsequently proved his idea.

Hoffmann–La Roche bought worldwide rights from Cetus for the PCR process, paying $300 million soon after it was invented. Roche then licensed the use of the technique to police department crime labs, research institutes, the military, and all others who had need for it.

Dr. Lai-Goldman said that when the company obtained the rights to PCR, it was brought to the new center that had been formed to further its development. Dr. Lai-Goldman said the work was very important because of the spread of HIV in the 1980s. She said that, at that time, everyone who contracted HIV died. Something was needed to bring it under control, and that was the aim of the Center for Molecular Biology and Pathology.

"This launched the facility," she said, and work there contributed to HIV being controlled. She said drugs received the credit for that, but she added that drugs would have been no good had it not been for the tests the center developed. Vital work was also done at the center with hepatitis, cystic fibrosis, and the human papillomavirus (HPV).

Dr. Lai-Goldman referred to this work as the birth of personalized medicine that would become so vital to patient care, and LabCorp was the first to do it.

By the 1990s Roche Biomedical Laboratories had acquired a number of properties across the nation, and in August 1990 the company underwent a program of geographic consolidation.

Labs in Sacramento, California, and Denver, Colorado, were sold to Unilab Corp for $41 million. Those labs were involved in clinical anatomical and cytology testing. Under terms of the sale, Roche Biomed retained its esoteric and specialty testing operations in those areas. Otherwise, this marked a withdrawal from the West Coast market at that time.

In May 1991 Roche Biomedical Laboratories made a new expansion by establishing its Consulting Physicians Network. The Roche subsidiary Roche Insurance Laboratory set up this operation to provide access to a medical insurance board-certified physician by underwriting companies that did not have a full-time staff physician. Physicians in this program performed a number of tasks, including the reading of EKGs and reviewing of files, all within one to two days. That network, according to company officials, complemented the lab's existing businesses and at the same time allowed the company to meet the changing needs of the insurance industry.

A Leader in the Clinical Laboratory Field

By the time 1991 came to an end, Roche Biomedical Laboratories was one of the major players in the clinical laboratory field. It was the second-largest medical testing company in the United States, with annual revenues of more than $600 million. There were more than 8,000 employees in some four hundred locations across the country.

Another major step came in February 1992 when Hoffmann–La Roche bought CompuChem Corporation, another North Carolina company, for $75 million. When

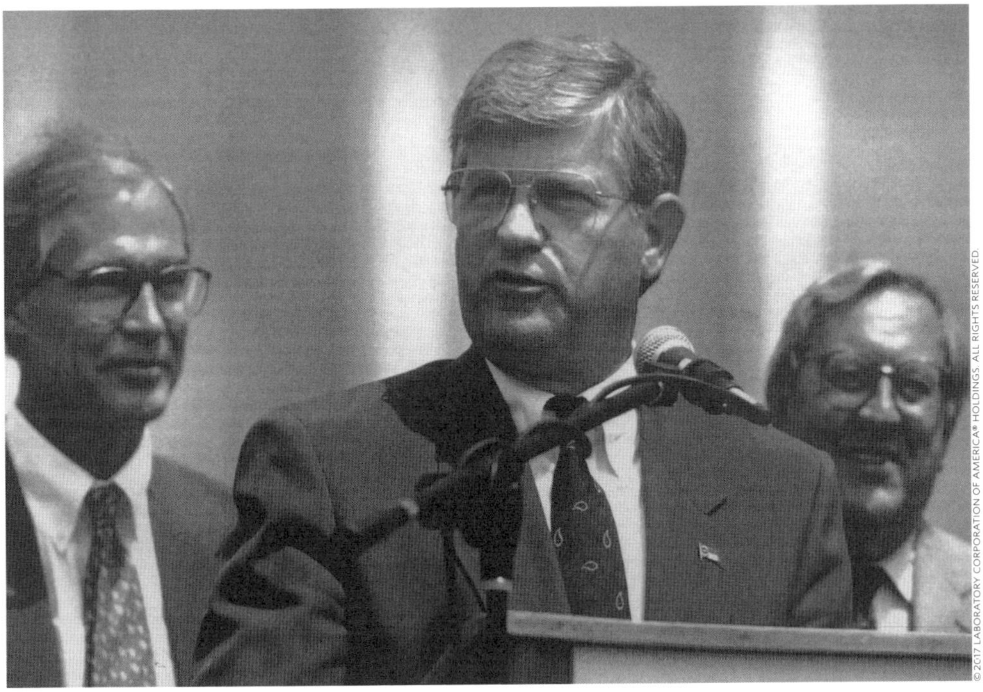

Gov. Jim Martin addresses crowd at York Court dedication in 1992. He is flanked on the left by Dr. Jim Powell and by Dick Murphy on the right.

that company was added to Roche Biomedical Laboratories, Roche became the second-largest drug-screening provider in the United States. The company already was second in paternity testing.

In May 1992 the company dedicated a 94,000-square-foot addition to the company's laboratory facilities on York Court in Burlington, making it one of the largest such laboratories in the world, with a total of 205,000 square feet. North Carolina Governor Jim Martin was present to help dedicate the new facilities, where some 850 people were employed, doing more than forty-three thousand forensic identification, cancer, allergy, AIDS, and other medical diagnostic tests on a daily basis.

In his remarks at the dedication that day, Governor Martin cited the company as "a model corporate citizen, committed to enhancing the state community through employment opportunities, as well as educational and other charitable initiatives." The company had more than 9,000 employees in more than five hundred locations across the nation at that time.

Thomas P. Mac Mahon, who was then president of the Roche Diagnostic Group, said "During these last ten years, RBL has become the largest and fastest-growing division" of the group. Dick Murphy, executive vice president of Roche US, also attended the presentation.

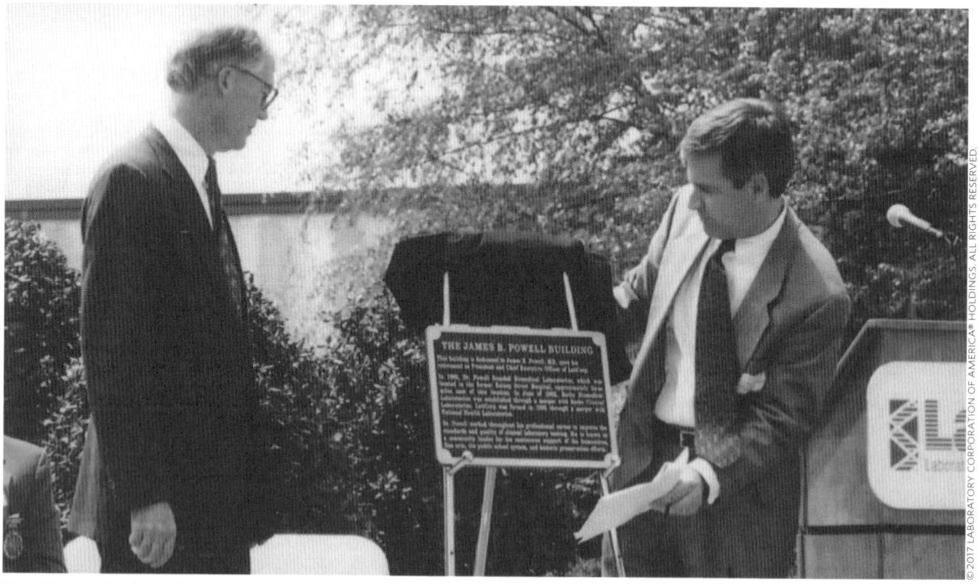

Brad Smith displays plaque honoring Dr. Jim Powell at dedication of the James B. Powell Building at York Court in 1992

Also speaking that day was Dr. Jim Powell, RBL's president. He gave credit for the company's success to its employees—"men and women of the highest caliber who bring to their work more than the usual quotient of professional excellence and personal commitment. They know that each test they perform may be critical to the health and well-being of someone's parent, child, or friend."

As the company grew and the list of services continued to increase, some elements emerged as not a good fit for RBL. One of those was the environmental division of CompuChem's operations. CompuChem had spent several million dollars developing its environmental testing products, but the expenses were too much for the size of the market. A major factor was uncertainty about state and local regulations—and uncertainty that left companies in doubt as to whether the processes were actually necessary. In view of this situation, the company sold off the environmental division of CompuChem in 1992.

As the company moved into the 1990s, it continued to adapt to the needs of its market, and a number of major technological advances were made, bringing new and favorable attention to Roche Biomedical Laboratories.

In 1992, one of the world's major health concerns dealt with the human immunodeficiency virus (HIV), and RBL was at the forefront of the effort to perform tests in dealing with it.

In July of that year, fifty-nine labs applied to the New York City Department of Health for approval to conduct tests for HIV. Roche Biomedical Laboratories in North Carolina and New Jersey was the first to gain approval. The company already had been approved by New York State.

HIV was a rapidly growing problem, and the company offered all available technologies for testing, including antibody tests and a special DNA test. That DNA test duplicated one strand of DNA millions of times in order to reveal the presence of the HIV virus. That DNA test was quite valuable in detecting HIV in newborn babies. Often those babies had not yet formed antibodies to the virus, so the test was a major step in combating that problem.

Another major development occurred in September 1992. At that time RBL introduced the first automated allergy test that used histamine levels to determine sensitivities in patients. In the past, this test had been labor-intensive and quite expensive, costing from $300 to $400 per antigen, and it also required a large blood sample. RBL's new product used leukocyte histamines, and it allowed physicians to run twenty-three tests for $115 while using only 2.6 milliliters of blood. In this test, allergens were mixed with the blood to see if a histamine reaction was produced.

About that same time, tuberculosis was making a resurgence in some areas, partially due to the advent of AIDS and new antibiotic-resistant strains of tuberculosis. The lab developed a new test to detect the tuberculosis bacterium in forty-eight hours, compared to three to six weeks in the past. This innovation was extremely important as it allowed treatment to begin much more quickly, shortening the time when the infected individual could contaminate others.

The polymerase chain reaction technology used in HIV and tuberculosis testing continued to be a development of ever-increasing importance for the company. It was used in a number of other tests, including those for HTLV-1 and HTLV-2, viruses believed to cause certain types of leukemia and lymphomas.

A new patient service center and laboratory was opened in Greenville, North Carolina, as 1992 ended. Two locations had served that area, and operations were combined into the new facility. Also at that time, the company was conducting financial and administrative operations in eleven different office buildings in downtown Burlington.

In the early 1990s, the company's Roche Image Analysis System (RIAS) was operating in the town of Elon. As Ernie Knesel had explained, work went on there through 1996 to improve its cervical cancer screening program, which used thin-layer slide preparations and computers to standardize the interpretation of Pap smear results. RIAS was soon to be spun off from RBL as a separate company, AutoCyte.

Further enhancements were made in DNA and paternity testing. By 1994 the company had a major share of the paternity testing market, which continued to grow.

CHAPTER SEVEN

Decentralization and Niche Businesses

WHEN BIOMEDICAL LABORATORIES WAS FIRST STARTED, it was one company located in Burlington, North Carolina. As the company grew, it did so concentrically, expanding out from its Burlington headquarters. This resulted in a centralized operation, with lab work, finance, customer service, sales, and marketing all directed and managed from one location. This centralized approach was continued even as the company expanded into Virginia, South Carolina, Tennessee, and Alabama.

Soon it became more difficult to manage the expanding company from one location due to logistics. Another factor was that local management generally knew best how to provide the unique service needs of the customer, and these requirements might differ in various locations. Another pressing need was to have service and financial accountability more identifiable on a local basis, starting with divisional heads on down into the various leadership roles within each division. The company soon began to reorganize by setting up these separate divisions geographically, with essentially all service and sales decisions being made at division headquarters.

The reference laboratories for more esoteric testing continued to be relatively centralized, for which the overnight airplane fleet was and continues to be used today. A few support functions also remained centralized in Burlington and the Research Triangle, which has continued into present times. Two large computer systems drive the company.

As the company grew to eventually become LabCorp, the divisions have been adjusted from time to time with different sizes and boundaries, but keeping with the concept of local decision making.

The need was also recognized for separate organizations to deal with integration of new technology into the company. These niche businesses were set up as separate companies, most of which had their own profit-and-loss statements and balance sheets prepared quarterly. The focus for each business was usually a new and specific area of the laboratory that was not traditional. The objective for forming these niche businesses in this way was to give employees and managers total responsibility for their efforts in a way that could be managed and measured as in any small company. They could hire people with very special skills and manage to specific objectives that were necessary for their unique niche.

The managers were also compensated for how well their individual businesses performed. This arrangement developed many entrepreneurs inside the parent company, who were known as "intrapreneurs." A number of these intrapreneurs have gone on to start their own businesses in the clinical laboratory and biotechnology world.

This niche business concept also gave more separation of a specific business within the organization at large. This business could then make mergers or even be divested as a separate and measurable business unit. A merger made by one of these businesses could be managed and evaluated very specifically and a determination made as to how much of the corporate resources should be devoted to growing the specific business. At one time there were fourteen of these businesses within Roche Biomedical Laboratories. In 1994 the ten niche businesses were as follows:

- Allergy testing—Computerized allergen tests, analysis, and treatment program.
- Ambulatory monitoring—Computer-assisted analysis of electrocardiograms and blood pressure.
- Clinical trials testing—Clinical laboratory testing for pharmaceutical companies conducting clinical research trials.
- Diagnostic genetics—Cytogenetic biochemical and molecular and genetic tests.
- Industrial hygiene testing—Analysis for potentially toxic substances in the workplace environment.

- Kidney stone analysis—Analysis of kidney stones that had been passed and the assessment of the risk of kidney stones.
- Oncology testing—Diagnosis and monitoring of certain cancer and treatment outcome predictions.
- Identity testing—Forensic identity testing used in connection with criminal proceedings and parentage evaluation services.
- Substance abuse testing—Urinalysis and breath and blood testing services for the detection of drugs of abuse.
- Veterinary testing—Clinical laboratory testing of animal specimens for veterinarians.

Ernie Knesel, one of those present on the first day of business in 1969, had stayed in operations over the years in addition to his other duties. When operations were decentralized he became the "king of the niches," a nickname given him by the employees. "I enjoyed that most of all," he said.

One of the niches was Kontron Electronics in Germany. "I was president while still a vice president for Biomedical" in 1989. He had become senior vice president of operations for Roche. Kontron had a large operation in California, he said, and after the acquisition, cuts were made. Kontron was moved to Burlington as Roche Image Analysis Systems (RIAS; later Images). More and more work came in for Images, he said, but when LabCorp was born in 1995, Images was not a part of the plan. He had to make a choice: RIAS or LabCorp. He stayed with "the little company," not LabCorp, and reported to Roche in Switzerland. His operation was on Orange Drive in Elon. Then in 1996, when Jim Powell left LabCorp he joined Knesel, and they were back together after a year. They renamed the company AutoCyte, with Powell as president and CEO. The company went public a few months later, and after two acquisitions it was renamed Tripath. Knesel said they developed a good product line, and later the company was sold to Beckton Dickinson of New Jersey for a substantial sum.

The formation of AutoCyte brought in the venture capitalists, and Knesel said that sometimes "working for venture capitalists can be a bit distasteful, but we made it a success." Yet when he left in 2000, "The venture capitalists threw me out." Most have now left the company themselves, he said.

In 2002 Knesel; his wife, Lynn; and their son, Bradley created a full-service laboratory in Greensboro in a historic textile mill building, the Revolution Mill, which was built in 1900. They served the areas of Greensboro, Raleigh, and southern Virginia.

"In 2011 Solstas made me an officer I could not refuse," and then a bit later, Quest bought Solstas.

In 2005 the Knesels, along with friend Jerry Denney, founded Synermed Select Partners Inc., which continues in operation today as Select Laboratory Partners (SLP). That company works with physicians, laboratories, and other clients to help them learn how to operate their own laboratories in a more efficient and better way.

In 2007 they created Select Labs in Manning, South Carolina, and it remains in operation today as well. Also in 2007 the Knesels and Denney created Cell Solutions to develop new technology related to Pap smears. This was the same work he had done at TriPath earlier. That operation continues today in Europe, Russia, China, and other areas.

Later in 2012 Knesel had a role in Infrared Laboratory Systems in Westfield, Indiana, a company begun by Craig Denney, Jerry Denney's son. Infrared deals with instruments and reagents.

By 1995 the clinical laboratory industry had hit hard times from a financial perspective. Medicare reimbursement levels had been cut severely, and the growing influence of managed care companies that set their own reimbursement schedules cut even more into lab companies' margins. In this atmosphere, lab companies began to consolidate and restructure. To keep up with the changes, companies were looking to run all their routine tests through operations that could process huge volumes of such tests with emphasis on quality, consistency, price, scope of tests, and convenience of service. Observers noted that those things would be the measures that would separate winners and losers.

Roche Biomedical Laboratories and three other laboratories began talks in the early 1990s about a possible merger that would do many of the things seen as necessary to keep RBL and the others from being among the losers.

In 1994, the four largest laboratories were Roche Biomedical Laboratories, National Health Laboratories, MetPath Laboratories, and SmithKline Beecham

Clinical Laboratories. For the previous two years, all had talked to each other about possible moves that would produce the largest one or two laboratory companies in the world. Dr. Jim Powell remembers that the merger process was not an easy thing.

"The merger of Roche Biomedical Laboratories and National Health Laboratories was easier said than done," he said.

RBL went in-depth discussions with three other labs; it was a lengthy and involved process.

Dr. Powell said that talks failed with SmithKline Beechman and Corning's MetPath, and discussions eventually began with National Health Laboratories (NHL), which was controlled by Ronald Perelman, the billionaire owner of MacAndrews & Forbes. He had made his fortune earlier in the cosmetics industry by owning Revlon and a number of other businesses.

According to Dr. Powell, the board at NHL also included Jim Maher, who had been CEO of National Health, and Linda Robinson, whose husband was the long-standing CEO of American Express. He said the Robinsons were social and business friends of Perelman. They and Maher, he said, had figured prominently in the North Carolina business world, with the sale of RJ Reynolds Nabisco and the move of its headquarters from Winston-Salem to Atlanta after the sale.

After long discussions, it was agreed to merge Roche Biomedical Laboratories and National Health Laboratories for a number of reasons. Dr. Powell explained that there was a large amount of overlap between the two companies, which he said "made this merger particularly attractive." It would be possible to combine operations in a number of territories with resulting efficiencies and savings. Dr. Powell said, "These synergies would help to justify the merger by improving earnings per share and avoiding dilution of earnings per share of the resulting company.... As the merger developed," he said, "Roche ended up with the controlling interest, and NHL shareholders received stock and a large cash payment."

In order to expedite the process of becoming a public company, the privately held RBL was technically merged into NHL, which was already publicly held.

Dr. Powell said, "Roche was in the driver's seat going forward due to its commanding ownership interests in the company. The agreement for the planned merger was consummated late in 1994 with due diligence taking place by both companies in the succeeding months, with the final merger in the spring of 1995."

As due diligence was being conducted to make way for the actual merger, Roche and NHL decision makers began deciding who would manage the proposed company going forward. A board of directors was formed, including Jim Maher from NHL. He was appointed to a one-year term as chairman of the board. He was succeeded a year later by Tom Mac Mahon from Roche's US organization.

Other board members included Drs. Andrew Wallace, David Skinner, and Jim Powell, as well as Linda Robinson for one year. Dr. Wallace was provost and CEO of Dartmouth Medical Center, and Dr. Skinner was CEO of the New York Hospital / Cornell Medical Center, which was soon to be merged with Columbia-Presbyterian in New York. Jean-Luc Bélingard, from the executive committee of Roche in Basel, Switzerland, was also on the board.

CHAPTER EIGHT

Laboratory Corporation of America

ON DECEMBER 13, 1994, THE DIRECTORS of Roche Biomedical Laboratories received an interoffice memo that included a certificate of action approving "the merger of the Corporation with and into National Health Laboratories Holdings Inc." The directors—Thomas Mac Mahon, H. F. Boardman, Dr. Jim Powell, Patrick J. Zenner and Martin F. Stadler—were asked to sign the documents, if they met with their approval, and return them to the secretary of the corporation. That four-page document, along with a certificate of action of stockholders, effectively began the legal process that created Laboratory Corporation of America.

The merger created the nation's largest operator of medical-test labs, with revenue of $1.7 billion, overtaking a unit of SmithKline Beecham PLC and Corning Inc.'s MetPath division. This new operation would include twenty thousand employees with thirty-nine labs that performed a variety of diagnostic tests for health-care providers.

Once again, observers of the lab industry saw this move as another step toward more large providers that could better control costs. It was more proof of the old adage that bigger is better.

Jean-Luc Bélingard, head of the Roche Diagnostics Division and member of the Roche Executive Committee in Basel, Switzerland, said at the time, "The combination of these two laboratory organizations will result in the creation of an industry leader. Our strong management team will be in a superior position to respond proactively to critical issues such as managed care. Roche thereby maintains its commitment to the clinical laboratory business and achieves a significantly enhanced strategic position in this field."

The merger process moved along quickly, and on April 28, 1995, the board of directors of the new corporation met in New York City to elect and appoint officers and to adopt an amended banking resolution. Directors present were James R. Maher, Thomas P. Mac Mahon, Jean-Luc Bélingard, Linda Gosden Robinson, and Bradford T. Smith, secretary. Dr. James B. Powell was present by telephone, and Drs. David B. Skinner and Andrew G. Wallace were absent. Those elected to management positions were as follows:

Dr. James B. Powell, president and chief executive officer
David C. Flaugh, executive vice president and chief operating officer
Bradford T. Smith, executive vice president, general counsel, and secretary
Timothy J. Brodnick, executive vice president, sales and marketing
Haywood D. Cochrane Jr., executive vice president and chief financial officer
John F. Markus, executive vice president, corporate compliance
Ronald B. Sturgill, executive vice president, information systems/operations
David C. Weavil, executive vice president and chief administrative officer
Robert Whalen, executive vice president, human resources
Wesley R. Elingburg, senior vice president, finance
Larry L. Leonard, executive vice president
Alvin Ezrin, vice president, law
David W. Gee, assistant secretary
John R. Erwin, assistant secretary

Senior vice presidents, with areas of duty, were

John Bergstrom, managed care
Woody Cook and Craig Dawson, operations
Lou Hadden and James P. Kilgore, operations
Gary Latimer, hospital joint ventures
J. Roland Mott and Jean S. Neff, operations

Gail S. Page, standardization and automation
Daniel R. Shoemaker, Fred A. Simpson, Timothy J. Smith, Michael F. Snyder, and Steve Stark, operations

Just a few days later, on May 1, 1995, James B. Maher, chairman of the board, and Dr. Jim Powell, president and CEO, sent a letter to clients that stated in part, "Today we completed the merger of National Health Laboratories Inc. and Roche Biomedical Laboratories Inc. The new company is Laboratory Corporation of America Holdings (or LabCorp), the largest clinical laboratory in the world in terms of revenue."

Clients were told, "Our daily operations will remain essentially the same," and "Our goal at LabCorp will be the same as it has always been: to provide you with the very best laboratory service possible."

A similar letter went to employees that same day, stating in part, "The ultimate success of LabCorp depends on your continuing dedication to excellence," and "Through your commitment, we can be confident of fulfilling our potential as Laboratory Corporation of America faces the challenges ahead."

National Health Laboratories was actually a wholly owned subsidiary of Revlon Holdings Inc. NHL was formed in the 1970s and after several acquisitions had assumed its position as one of the "Big Four." By 1993 it had grown to $761 million in revenue.

The chief financial officer of the new company was Haywood D. Cochrane Jr., a familiar name in the Burlington operations. He had previously served in that capacity in Burlington.

In 1994, just prior to the merger, National Health Laboratories had acquired Allied Clinical Laboratories in Tennessee. Cochrane had been president and CEO of Allied, and he became vice chairman of NHL. Before that he had been with Biomedical Laboratories, having moved there from Wachovia Bank. He was chief financial officer at Biomedical, and he led the initial public offering when Biomedical became a public company in 1979 and changed its name to Biomedical Reference Laboratories.

Five years later Cochrane had, with the backing of venture money, bought Allied Clinical Laboratories in Nashville, Tennessee. Just as he had done at Biomedical Laboratories, he did some financial cleanup work and then led it to becoming publicly owned. It was soon sold to National Health Laboratories. It was only a few months until NHL joined Roche Biomedical to form LabCorp, where Cochrane became chief financial officer.

Cochrane said Jim Powell had to deal with major cultural differences in this merger process, but he was a person "who did things the right way."

"Jim is the most upright and honest person I know," he said, adding that he worked through difficult situations at times to resolve problems related to those different cultures. "Every transition was another culture shock, and he did a great job" in handling them, Cochrane said.

He also said that Powell was absolutely steadfast that the headquarters of the company would stay in Burlington every time there was a merger. That was always the "deal breaker," Cochrane said. If Burlington was not going to be the headquarters site, then there would be no deal.

One day in the early years, "We almost went out of business," Cochrane said. It was a Saturday in May, he remembered, and a new computer had been shipped to Burlington. It was being moved into the facility on a system of rails when suddenly it slipped off those rails.

"Jim and I held it on until we could get help. Had it fallen, we would have been out of business."

"We had really good people" in the company, and they were quite frugal as well, Cochrane recalled.

"We did not want to waste money. Jim is frugal, but I am more frugal," he laughed. "When traveling we stayed two to a room, we flew coach," and he remembered an incident with a cab driver in New York City when he was with Jim and Ed Powell in the cab. At the destination Cochrane said he would take care of the tip. "I gave the driver a seventy-five-cent tip, and he threw it back at me," declaring that if that was all I would give him, he did not want it." The others felt he might have carried his frugality a bit too far that day.

Cochrane went back to Nashville in 1997 to form another company, only to return to Burlington in 2002.

The merger between Roche Biomedical Laboratories and National Health Laboratories was good news for Burlington and for North Carolina. At the time, there were about seventeen hundred Roche-Biomedical Laboratories employees in Burlington and between six thousand and seven thousand across North Carolina. Those numbers would grow significantly in the future, as this was a major economic boost for the entire area.

But not everyone was happy.

CHAPTER NINE

Burlington Is Headquarters

A HEADLINE IN THE *San Diego (CA) Union-Tribune* on the day of the announcement read, “Lab Merger Will Create a Giant, but Not Here.”

The headquarters of National Health Laboratories was located in La Jolla near San Diego, and the story said the headquarters of the new company would “in all probability” be located in Burlington, North Carolina, home of RBL. Operations would remain in San Diego, but “there may be ‘some consolidation’ of employees in coming weeks and months.”

Jim Powell was serving as CEO in Burlington, and he was an MD who was also a pathologist. Roche wanted someone with business and scientific credentials in charge. Also in Powell’s favor was the fact that he had served as CEO of a public company earlier at Biomedical Reference Laboratories, and a professional team was in place with which Roche was comfortable.

So Burlington, North Carolina, a city of fewer than fifty thousand people, became the national headquarters of what would become an S&P 500 company and a world leading life sciences company. That was in no small part due to the role that Jim Powell had played in the company from the very beginning.

For those who were surprised, it did not take long to realize what a good choice Burlington was. Burlington sits almost in the middle of North Carolina. Interstates 40 and 85 run right through the city limits, and one of the finest business airports in the state is located on the southern edge of the city.

Greensboro, High Point, and Winston-Salem are but a few miles to the west, and the Research Triangle is a few miles to the east, anchored by Raleigh, Durham, and Chapel Hill. Raleigh is home to North Carolina State University, Durham to Duke University, and Chapel Hill to the University of North Carolina.

In Greensboro are UNC-Greensboro, North Carolina A&T State University, Greensboro College, Guilford College, and Bennett College.

But "right across the street" from LabCorp's York Court campus is the campus of Elon University. Elon is rated as a national leader in many areas of education; it is a perennial leader in study abroad programs and has been ranked for several years in many other categories, including "the prettiest university campus" in the nation.

LabCorp and Elon University have cooperated over the years to develop numerous management training courses for LabCorp managers.

In determining the management of the new company, Dr. Powell said that negotiators had compromised with the best of intentions to try to incorporate all of the talents from all of the senior management from both companies.

"For much of the first year," he said, "the new board insisted that every effort should be made to accomplish the merger goals with this unwieldy management group. This view proved to be costly, time-consuming, stressful, and unsuccessful."

The initial senior management team of the company included Dr. Jim Powell as CEO with senior vice presidents Haywood Cochrane, Brad Smith, and David Weavil from RBL; and David Flaugh, Tim Brodnick, and Bob Whelan from NHL.

Dr. Powell said it became apparent to him and others very early that this team was not going to be successful. He said the two companies had been managed very differently by two totally different groups for many years. There were also certain residual feelings of hostility from many years of being primary competitors among the four largest laboratories—including lawsuits. NHL had actually been the first competitor that Biomedical Laboratories had encountered on its first day of operation.

As Dr. Powell explained, "The mechanics of the merger were by their nature bound to create resentments in all quarters of the new company. Much of the synergy was by necessity accomplished by combining laboratories, with the resulting loss of jobs by those whose entity did not survive. LabCorp was now a public company with many shareholders that had expectations regarding these anticipated efficiencies and resulting cost savings that had been used to justify the merger from the beginning."

As soon as the merger was consummated, the combination of various overlapping laboratory operations began in earnest. For example, in North Carolina, LabCorp now had a large presence in Burlington—earlier owned by RBL—and also another large operation in Winston-Salem—previously owned by NHL. The proximity made it possible to essentially eliminate one of the operations—in this case, the NHL operation. Similar operations had to be undertaken on a national basis, and the determination of the survivors began in earnest. Adding to the stress was the fact that all this had to be accomplished by December 31, 1996.

Dr. Powell said that a territory would be evaluated and the pros and cons would be determined for the respective RBL and NHL operations. One advantage, he said, of combining into previous RBL locations was the centralized computer system that the company and its predecessors had always employed. NHL had made acquisitions of various laboratories but had generally not consolidated their information technology. This approach, he explained, resulted in their having mostly stand-alone operations without the efficiencies and quality controls afforded by centralized computing.

Since RBL people were in charge, there was a natural inclination to go with managers, employees, and laboratory operations that were proven entities to them. Dr. Powell said that the NHL alumni became increasingly wary and suspicious as time went by, and in their view their position was deteriorating. The three senior NHL managers were gone voluntarily in the first year, partly due to a large bonus they were to receive if they left in that time period.

The merger activity stressed management, who were responsible for getting those changes in place. Adding to the stress, management was blamed for the job loss itself.

Dr. Jim Kilgore remembers a meeting in Washington, DC, when the name of the new company was announced. There had been a contest within the company, and managers in Roche Biomed and National Health Labs came together for the first time.

"They [NHL] flew in first class and stayed in suites," Kilgore remembers, and the Roche people flew in coach and stayed two to a room. "Jim was tight and he expected you to be," Kilgore said.

That was some indication of the cultural difference between the two groups, he remembers. He said that in one meeting a Roche manager got up and left, saying, "I can't deal with these people."

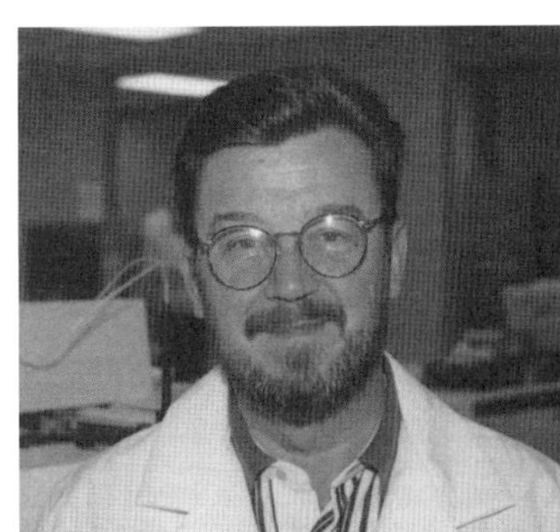

Dr. Jim Kilgore

On the day of the announcement, everyone went into a huge room that looked a lot like a sports arena. NHL people were on one side "in their coats and ties," and Roche Biomed had the other side. Down in the middle was Jim Powell with other officials when the page was flipped on a big easel to display the name "LabCorp" for the first time.

Kilgore was head of microbiology with Diagnostics Laboratory in Charlotte when it became a part of Biomedical Reference Laboratories in 1981. That laboratory had been in direct competition with BRL. Kilgore and Ron Sturgill worked there together, and after the acquisition, Sturgill moved to Burlington and Kilgore stayed in Charlotte to run the RBL labs in Charlotte, Columbia, and Charleston. He did not move to Burlington until 1989, when he and Danny Shoemaker ran the Elon operation. The Atlantic Division was split then; Kilgore ran one section, and Shoemaker, the other. Later Shoemaker transferred to Alabama, and Kilgore took over the entire operation.

Kilgore said Diagnostic's merger with Biomed went well. "We knew each other," although they were competitors, and "we were friends."

The union with Roche went well also, he said.

As for the Roche-NHL merger that created LabCorp, Kilgore said, "NHL was more sales-oriented, and Jim Powell was more oriented on service." It finally turned out okay, he said. "They had sales, and we had science—and then it took off."

"The basic success came in Jim Powell's leadership and the people he surrounded himself with," Kilgore explained. People worked hard for him as well, because "we did not want to let him down."

Kilgore said he had wanted to be a doctor but did not have the money to pursue that career, but when he was running the laboratory in Elon, "It was like being a doctor on speed." He could do fifty or more tests per day. "We did not see the patients but we helped them."

Kilgore retired in 2008 as a senior vice president after what he described as "a heck of a ride."

Genomics and Personalized Medicine

In the years that followed the merger, LabCorp continued to expand its esoteric and specialty laboratory testing. Genomics, anatomic pathology, and personalized medicine were focuses of the company.

In May 1995 LabCorp announced plans to expand its medical testing facilities in Research Triangle Park in the Raleigh–Durham–Chapel Hill area. A new 92,000-square-foot laboratory facility was planned as an expansion of the company's two existing labs there already, one of which was completed only four years earlier.

Whit Morrow, facilities chief for the company, said one of the labs there already concentrated on drug testing while the second dealt with specialty tests, such as DNA, genetics, and oncology. The proximity of the labs to Raleigh-Durham International Airport allowed for quick tests for clients. Tests for the labs are flown into the airport from all over the country every night.

In August of that same year the company announced plans to purchase a large hosiery plant in downtown Burlington. Kayser-Roth Hosiery had vacated the 176,000-square-foot building, and LabCorp planned to use historical tax credits for renovations. The building was an integral part of the Burlington hosiery industry in the 1930s and later. This was another step in the company's plans for preserving elements of the city's history.

Two months later the company announced plans for a new 70,000-square-foot facility on its York Court site in Burlington. The $3.5 million building was built on twenty acres of additional land purchased in 1991 and would allow a new entrance to the site off West Front Street in Burlington. The facility would house the cytology lab, which tests Pap smears; the paternity lab; the histology lab; and a section for bone marrow testing and registration.

The year 1996 was highlighted by major transactions that made the LabCorp name a bigger player in the hospital industry. The company signed a three-year laboratory management contract with Nyack Hospital in Nyack, New York. A similar contract was signed with the Kentucky Division of Columbia/RCA Healthcare Corporation, one of the state's largest health-care services. The Kentucky contract paved the way for a major national contract signed in early 1996.

Jim Powell, in his message to shareholders that year, had some prophetic words about the future of the laboratory industry:

> The industry as a whole will continue to be transformed by stricter reimbursement policies, adverse utilization trends, and heightened competition spurred by government cutbacks and by the growth of managed care, physician alliances, and affiliations between consumer groups.

But LabCorp, he said, "is prepared for a tough, difficult environment."

He was correct in his assessment of the industry in general, as things would change dramatically in the years to come for the reasons he cited, and he was correct also that LabCorp indeed was prepared for that environment. LabCorp's history is filled with innovative programs that made improvements for its clients, and while those programs have made headlines for the company, other programs were developed for the company's workforce.

In February 1996 it was announced that LabCorp was partnering with another Alamance County industry to provide a health-care benefit system for employees. Glen Raven Mills, an internationally known textile operation, has its main facility within two miles of LabCorp operations at York Court. Formed in 1880, Glen Raven Mills was a major player in textiles and hosiery—they patented panty hose—and then moved into outdoor specialty fabrics. Their Sunbrella awning fabrics are known around the world.

The two companies formed a nonprofit organization in which employers contracted with hospitals and physicians for discount rates for medical services. The Piedmont Health Care Coalition Inc. was designed to hold down costs and improve the quality of care for employees. The coalition developed hospital and physician networks in Burlington, Greensboro, and Chapel Hill, with others to come later. President Gregory A. Walters, a former health benefits manager at LabCorp, said, "Rather than waiting for the government to mandate health-reform measures, this new health coalition is taking an active role in stimulating community-based reform initiatives."

Later that year the company initiated an employee stock purchase plan. Employees could purchase company stock at a 15 percent discount and pay no commissions on plan purchases, with access to discounted transaction fees.

By June 1996 LabCorp had grown to a network of thirty-one major laboratories with some fifteen hundred branches, patient service centers, and STAT laboratories operating in forty-eight states. At that time the most frequent tests performed were blood chemistry analysis, urinalysis, blood cell counts, Pap smears, AIDS tests, microbiology cultures procedures, and alcohol and other substance abuse tests. In August of that same year LabCorp placed nineteenth in a ranking of the state's seventy-five largest public companies.

A longtime employee, Wesley R. Elingburg, became senior vice president, chief financial officer, and treasurer on October 25, 1996.

Elingburg had been with Roche Biomedical Laboratories for fifteen years and had been a member of the management committee since the merger. He succeeded Haywood D. Cochrane Jr., who continued as a consultant.

At the same time, four other appointments were made to the management committee: Larry Leonard, executive vice president, Southwest and West Divisions; William M. Meihlan, senior vice president, chief information officer; Steven R. Stark, executive vice president, alliances and sales coordination; and Ronald B. Sturgill, executive vice president, human resources and South Atlantic Division.

Government vs. Laboratories

In November 1996 a long-running legal case between LabCorp and the federal government regarding the company's billing practices came to a conclusion. The two parties "agreed to disagree," and the situation was brought to an end. In the early 1990s the Justice Department and the Federal Bureau of investigation had begun reviewing the entire health-care industry. At issue was the way in which the government was being billed for laboratory tests by private and commercial labs as well as hospitals. There was a conviction on the part of the Office of the Inspector General and the Department of Health and Human Services that the government was paying too much for laboratory testing, but the government did not have a clear case for attacking the problem.

As early as November 1990, National Health Labs became aware of a grand jury inquiry relating to its pricing practices. This was being conducted by the US Attorney for the Southern District of California. An assistant DA in San Diego had reckoned that physicians were being "induced" by laboratories to over-order laboratory tests—despite the fact that the physicians were the gatekeepers for ordering tests. Labs cannot order tests. That case was settled in 1992.

The government also contended that laboratories were giving discounts to physicians for lab work that the physician was paying for and not extending the discounts to Medicare and Medicaid. The government also argued that labs were including more tests in the profiles than the doctors needed for a simple profile, and that the doctors were using the same ordering patterns for patients that they billed as for Medicare and Medicaid patients.

The 1990–1992 case against NHL claimed that the company had included the HDL cholesterol test and a test for ferritin in its basic profile for the physicians without charging any additional amount for these tests. Because the testing labs billed the government directly for these tests, and each of the tests had an additional payment code, Medicare would be charged additional amounts for the HDL and ferritin tests. The government's position in the case was that the testing lab had a duty to tell the doctor that the tests were going to cost the government more, regardless of whether they cost the doctors more, in which case the doctor might have decided not to order them. The government claimed it had evidence from doctors who said that because the additional tests were part of a panel, they were not aware the government would pay more for them.

Physicians had negotiated pricing with labs for years. Medicare, on the other hand, always paid according to a fixed-fee schedule for selected panels and tests. Medicare paid the same way for drugs. The NHL case was settled in 1992 without going to court. The general feeling was that most laboratories had little choice but to try to settle rather than litigate the government's allegations.

That 1992 settlement was not the end of it, however. Government charges were soon to be expanded to other independent labs and hospital labs. By 1993, subpoenas from the Office of the Inspector General had gone out to National Health Laboratories, Corning (MetPath), SmithKline Beecham, Unilabs, Damon, Roche Biomedical, Allied, Nichols Institute, and essentially all of the major commercial laboratories.

Hospital labs were also being charged with improper billing, and by October 1996, ten Ohio hospitals had settled claims that they overcharged the federal Medicare and Medicaid programs for outpatient lab tests. The Ohio Hospital Association and the American Hospital Association then sued HHS secretary Donna Shalala, alleging that the US government was improperly seeking cash penalties for alleged overbilling by at least 150 hospitals in Ohio alone. Both the hospital groups maintained that member hospitals weren't told of the new billing standards until 1993 and that they should not be forced to pay for the government's own negligence in failing to tell them.

On another note, by December 1996 the US Justice Department had quietly settled with 1,000 hospitals in an unusual "gentleman's agreement" for repeated double billing for outside services. Daniel Rubin, in an article for Knight-Ridder News Service on December 6, 1996, reported that the agreements were that federal officials would not announce the civil settlements if the hospitals paid the money willingly.

Independent clinical laboratories were not offered a gentleman's agreement, as they were publicly characterized as under investigation by the Justice Department for "fraud and abuse."

The Office of the Inspector General also charged that laboratories did not inform the physicians of how Medicare and Medicaid paid for tests. However, the Medicare and Medicaid fee schedules paying for laboratory work were public information and available to physicians.

A number of the larger profiles offered by RBL did include some of the fourteen tests that the government claimed were being added to the profiles. The company, however, also offered the basic profiles without any added tests that the government was wanting the physicians to see. The physicians were free to order those basic profiles for their Medicare and Medicaid patients.

As laboratories became more capable over the years and more was learned about the value of laboratory testing, there was, according to Dr. Powell, a natural inclination to build bigger panels and profiles for physicians who understood how to interpret and use tests that went beyond the basic panel. A good example, he said, would be the HDL cholesterol or "good cholesterol" test that brought complaints from the government. It is a test that is extremely important for knowledgeable physicians in managing lipids in the blood. Dr. Powell said it was the job of the lab's salespeople to educate the physicians on the value of laboratory testing and to increase the utilization of those valuable tools in health care.

There was no program or intention of having salespeople try to induce physicians to abuse the Medicare or Medicaid system of reimbursement, Dr. Powell said. In addition, he said, RBL always maintained the ability of the physician to order the basic profile for Medicare and Medicaid patients. Nonetheless, the government took the position that offering the basic panels was not sufficient because the laboratories failed to tell the doctors that the government would pay more for the larger panels, even though the doctors who were billed directly did not pay more.

Eventually, financial settlements totaling well over a billion dollars were made by hundreds of clinical laboratories in the United States to settle mostly civil lawsuits. LabCorp paid $187 million to settle with the government.

Dave Weavil had been with the company since the 1970s and had been part of its growth with the Roche acquisition and in the LabCorp formation as well. He was an accountant with the Peat Marwick Mitchell CPA firm in Greensboro after his 1974 graduation from the University of North Carolina in business and accounting.

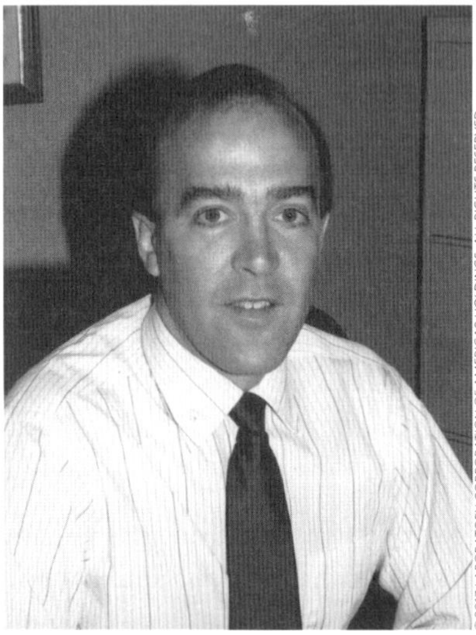

David Weavil

One of the clients he served was Biomedical Laboratories. It was not long until he was part of Biomedical himself, serving as chief financial officer. Weavil was there during the time the company went public, and then as it became Roche Biomedical, serving in a variety of capacities, including senior vice president and chief operating officer.

After a successful career with BRL, RBL and LabCorp, Weavil moved to the West Coast and served as CEO of two laboratories there before moving back to the North Carolina Piedmont in 2007. He and a financial backer later bought Spectrum Labs in Greensboro, one of Ernie Knesel's operations. Weavil served as CEO of Spectrum Labs, competing with LabCorp. In 2016 he was still in the industry as a consultant.

"Jim [Powell] and I had lots of fun times. He is a true visionary. He took action on a concept in 1969 when there were no large regional labs. He said, 'We will take the mom-and-pop labs in local towns'" and make a big one. According to Weavil, Powell also said, "Let's put logistics out there and lower the costs," and Weavil said, "That's exactly what we did."

Weavil had some ideas about the future of the industry, noting that laboratory testing will always be critical to the delivery of good health care.

Also, he said, he fears there will be less development of high esoteric testing due to the costs involved and in the regulations of the FDA.

Weavil predicted that testing will get better, and there will be fewer hospital systems, with similar numbers of health care organizations. "They will be paid on the value they bring to the patient.... There will be far fewer providers, but they will be a lot larger," he said.

Weavil also said that patients today are often routed to many different areas for treatment, but in the future he believes patients with chronic health diseases will be managed day to day—getting their meds, doing their rehab, and being monitored at all times in order to keep them in the best possible condition.

One of the things most critical to the merger that had formed LabCorp was computer consolidation.

Pat Frele remembers that problem well, as it was her duty to help resolve it. She said that when the merger took place, all the entities that came together were using different systems. It did not take long, she said, to see that the situation was just not going to work.

For instance, if an electrical storm knocked out systems at one location, it was not possible to divert work to a system in another location. She became part of a conversion team that went all over the country converting laboratory and financial services to be compatible.

"Every week I was on a plane Monday morning and back Thursday night" to work on conversion issues. Frele recalls, "That work was very rewarding. We believed that we contributed to the creation of LabCorp" by getting operations in many different areas "all on the same page."

Robert E. Mittlestaedt Jr. was a director at the time. He was vice dean of the Wharton School of Business at the University of Pennsylvania. He said that in the late 1990s, after the merger that formed LabCorp, the company had many different billing systems. He said there was much needed work to be done in billing and collecting, and that it was needed for survival.

"We were just not making much money," he said. "We were doing great lab testing," but there was a lot of work to be done in the "blocking and tackling"—the basic parts of the business.

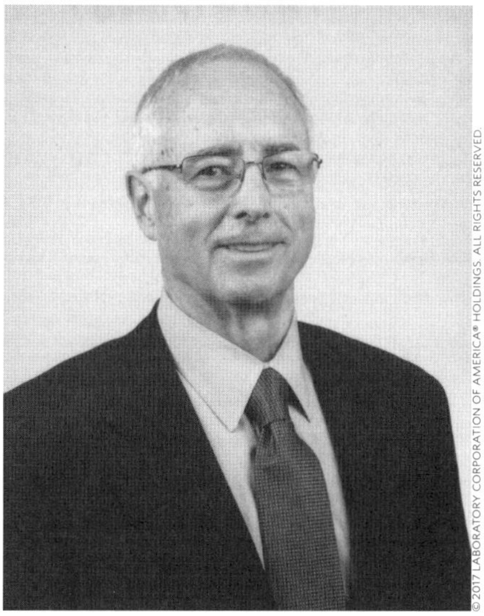

Robert E. Mittlestaedt Jr.

Things were so bad that the New York Stock Exchange was threatening to delist LabCorp. On June 1, 1996, the price of LabCorp stock was $19.06 per share with a market cap of $937 million. One year later, the share price was $7.19, with a market cap of only $353 million.

The stock fell even more in the next year, with a price of $5.31 on June 1, 1998, and a market cap of $265 million. Ten years later, things were much better, with a stock price of $59.80 and a market cap of $7.468 billion.

This period with both the government investigation and the merger with NHL had been perhaps the darkest in the company's history.

Wesley Elingburg said that the federal investigation explained "the worst of times," and the NHL merger and its problems were right behind it. The entire industry was in upheaval all across the nation, he said, and the NHL merger had been particularly difficult. He said the two companies were being operated in totally different ways, but that "Jim Powell did an incredible job getting the two companies together for the success of LabCorp."

All this affected the financial picture, and Elingburg said he remembers that, at one time, "There was a serious discussion as to whether we could make the payroll." But "everyone stuck with it, and the strategic plan [to come later] worked."

Elingburg said Jim Powell did an incredible job with his vision, and Tom Mac Mahon, who followed Powell, was also a visionary and took the company to even greater levels.

Elingburg retired in 2005 but continued to be busy as managing partner of the Greensboro Grasshoppers, the professional baseball team in Greensboro, and as a trustee at both Elon and Western Carolina Universities. He also serves on the board of the Hospice of Alamance/Caswell Counties.

The "worst of times" as referenced by Elingburg was a period of twenty months stretching from May 1995 to December 31, 1996. Dr. Jim Powell summarized those twenty months as a stressful time, a period that had been agreed upon as the time frame to realize all of the synergies expected when RBL and NHL agreed to merge. He said the expected cost savings from the synergies, mostly from the overlaps of the two companies, had been a great part of the justification for the merger.

"To realize the savings, much was expected from managers in the operations, sales, and information systems areas of the company. This resulted in the new company having to turn inwards for twenty months to accomplish the merger, he explained.

Thousands of people lost their jobs, and operations managers were charged with accomplishing this workforce reduction as redundant operations were "rationalized" or "right-sized." Hundreds of sales and marketing managers and representatives took on the task of leading current clients of the two companies through the process of change. The information systems staff had the difficult job of converting the many laboratory and billing systems existing in the NHL environment to the central systems that RBL had developed. This move was necessary for efficiency and quality control in the company's laboratory and financial areas. It was a crucial first step in standardizing laboratory procedures in all of the laboratories that would constitute LabCorp going forward.

This work was accomplished in twenty months and resulted in a $120-million-per-year savings for LabCorp that would flow straight to the bottom line for years to come.

"This turning inward," Dr. Powell said, "accomplished great savings, but it also resulted in lack of new sales during that period, and many onetime costs were incurred especially in the IS area."

The government settlement affected the laboratory industry from 1992 into 1997 as the various laboratories dealt with payments. LabCorp finalized its settlement in late 1996. Interestingly enough, there were no reports of laboratories or laboratory companies going directly to court over the government's claims. This was primarily due to fears of being excluded from government programs during the discovery and litigation process. There were several instances in which trade groups or lobbyists lodged complaints and instituted legal actions.

The government settlement would also require the laboratory industry to reconfigure test offerings reimbursed by the government, primarily in the panels and profiles that were offered. All these activities required a large amount of cash to consummate. The merger with NHL had also required considerable cash to pay the NHL shareholders.

This financial drain would soon require the establishment of a large debt "facility," which required borrowing over $1 billion from eleven national and international banks.

By that time LabCorp was the top employer in North Carolina in research/testing, with 4,240 employees, and that same number of employees ranked fifty-third overall in all categories of employment.

CHAPTER TEN

Jim Powell Makes a Change

JIM POWELL WAS NOT COMPLETELY HAPPY with his role as CEO in this type of corporate environment. He had always enjoyed his previous CEO roles at Biomedical Laboratories, Biomedical Reference Laboratories, and Roche Biomedical Laboratories. He said he had always been allowed a great deal of autonomy in those previous situations with very little interference from the boards of the first two companies or from Roche management in Nutley, New Jersey, during the RBL tenure.

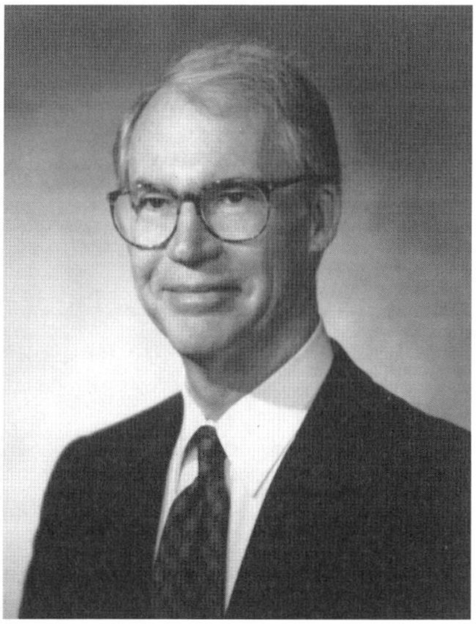

Dr. James B. Powell

The LabCorp situation was different.

"This new arrangement proved to be quite difficult, with countervailing opinions from certain of the original board members. In addition, the new job was to serve as CEO of a very large public company with initial revenues of $1.6 billion and over twenty thousand employees. It was an honor to be CEO of a public Fortune 500 company that was now one of the two largest laboratories in the country. One might think that this should have been viewed as the pinnacle of a career, but this position was becoming primarily a financial job. It required dealing on a constant basis with the many investor groups as one of the primary job descriptions, which was not appealing."

In the spring of 1996, as the merger activities were well under way, Powell met with Tom Mac Mahon, who was soon to become chairman of the new company. They discussed future plans and the progress of the merger. Then the conversation turned to what Dr. Powell wanted to do in the future. There was solid backing from the company if he wanted to stay on in his position, but in his words, "There was no joy or fun in the job any longer."

The conversation then moved to something that was of great interest to him—something far more entrepreneurial and technical than what lay before him at LabCorp.

There had been a development project at RBL for several years called Roche Imaging Analysis Systems (RIAS), as Ernie Knesel described earlier. The goal was to develop a thin-layer technology and imaging system to greatly improve cytology testing for cervical cancer. Powell and Knesel had worked together to get the initial Biomedical Laboratories off the ground, and Powell had great confidence in Knesel. Knesel was in charge of innovation at RBL, and he had led the RIAS development project.

Dr. Powell was also totally aware of the great potential for this effort as a separate company. He realized that the larger entity would need to allow the spinoff independence for the best success. Dr. Powell told Mac Mahon that a spinoff of this company would interest him if he could take a leadership role and become one of the primary owners.

The RIAS spinoff opportunity was agreed to at the spring meeting in 1996. Dr. Powell committed then and there to transitioning to this new opportunity after the merger consolidations were complete in six to eight months, at the end of calendar year 1996.

Formation of the new company, named AutoCyte, began in the spring of 1996, and it was publicly announced on November 25, 1996. Dr. Powell left the management of LabCorp on December 31, 1996, but remained as a director. He immediately joined the new company.

AutoCyte had two venture capital firms, Ampersand Ventures based in Massachusetts and the Sprout Group from California. These two groups combined with Roche interests and Dr. Powell to become the primary owners.

The new company initially focused on women's health—specifically on the early detection of cervical cancer. The initial products were AutoCyte PREP, which was a monolayer slide preparation system, and AutoCyte SCREEN, a computer-based imaging system for screening the monolayer slides to detect cancer and precancerous cells.

This new system's intended use was to replace the single best cancer detection system ever invented, the fifty-year-old Pap smear. Dr. Powell had spent a year in a fellowship at the New York Hospital / Cornell Medical Center in New York City in the cytology lab of Dr. Georgios Papanikolaou, who had developed that test. This past experience was an added inducement for Dr. Powell to be involved in the continuation of Dr. Georgios Papanikolaou's work.

The FDA required a premarket approval (PMA) for the new test. A premarket approval is the most vigorous scrutiny that the FDA can give a new medical device or test. It is required when there is no existing equivalent or predicate device.

The PMA required AutoCyte to conduct a double-blind study of ten thousand women to prove that detection rates were superior to what the traditional Pap smear had accomplished over the previous fifty years.

The AutoCyte study was conducted in the United States, South Africa, and South Vietnam. The latter sites were necessary in order to find locations with a higher incidence of cervical cancer. The Pap smear had been so successful in the United States over the previous fifty years that cervical cancer rates in the Western world were quite low.

The AutoCyte development was an innovative, proven improvement on health care for women worldwide. There was a successful initial public offering a few months after formation of the company. AutoCyte was later sold to Becton-Dickenson (BD), a large health-care conglomerate, and BD continues to expand the use of the new technology with improved cancer detection rates.

Thomas P. Mac Mahon had become chairman of the board, president, and chief executive officer of LabCorp in 1997 following a career in the Hoffmann–La Roche organization dating back to 1969. He held positions of increasing responsibility over the years in pharmaceutical marketing, public affairs, and strategic planning. He had been responsible since 1988 for the management of all US operations of the company's diagnostic business, and as a member of the executive committee of Hoffmann–La Roche, he also had oversight of Roche Biomedical Laboratories from 1988 to 1995.

Mac Mahon was senior vice president of Hoffmann–La Roche from 1993 to January 1997, and president of Roche Diagnostics Group and a member of the executive committee from 1988 to December 1996. He had received a BS in marketing from

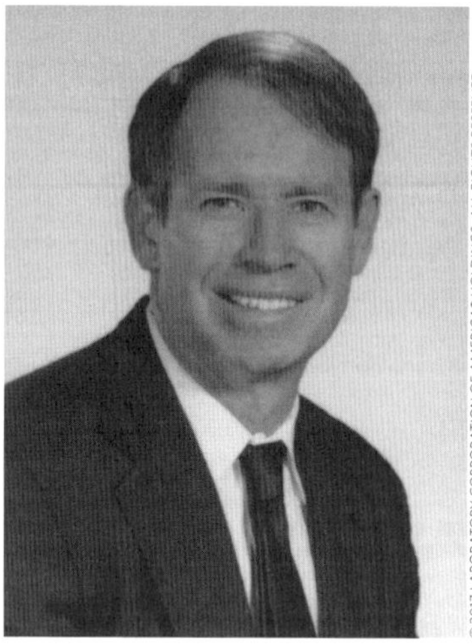

Tom Mac Mahon

Saint Peter's University and an MBA in marketing from Fairleigh Dickinson University.

Mac Mahon made his first report to the stockholders in early 1997. It was a positive one, reflecting the merged company's major plans for the future. Mac Mahon reported that the merger had brought "annualized run rate cost savings of approximately $120 million, exceeding our initial estimates of $80–$90 million." He also reported that the company had established a number of partnerships with health-care provider organizations, adding six new alliance agreements, "representing approximately $20 million in annual sales."

The CEO further noted that the emergence of preventative medicine as the driving force in health care had raised clinical laboratories to unprecedented prominence.

"Our past president, Dr. James B. Powell, was a pioneer in building this vital industry, helping to establish LabCorp as an industry leader."

At that point, LabCorp had about thirteen hundred varieties of tests in common use, and Mac Mahon said that in ten to fifteen years, that number was likely to double. Introduction of new tests would continue to be the company's major focus, along with the administration of those tests to offer maximum value to patients and health-care providers.

The federal government was getting more active in health care, affecting everyone in the medical professions from doctors to clinics, hospitals, managed care facilities, and medical testing laboratories.

As LabCorp had noted in its 1996 annual report, "In the past several years, the company's business has been affected by significant government regulation, price competition, and increased influence of managed care organizations resulting from payers' efforts to control the costs, utilization, and delivery of health care services." All this had a negative impact on the company's profitability.

"Changes were occurring as well," the annual report continued, with a shift away from traditional fee-for-service medicine to managed-cost health care. Managed care providers were contracting with a limited number of clinical laboratories and negotiating discounts to lab fees in an effort to control costs.

This situation was cutting into prices and "has negatively impacted the company's operating margins." Medicare, Medicaid, and other insurers were working to reduce costs and delivery of health services.

LabCorp looked for substantial savings in operations. The merger had a positive effect on costs, and ways were sought to improve profitability with the consolidation of certain operations and the elimination of redundant expenses.

This was not an issue just for 1996 but would be a major consideration in years to come as government regulations and a shift to managed care would bring increasing pressure on the clinical laboratory industry.

Despite all the negative pressures, however, LabCorp managed to increase net sales in 1996 by $178.7 million to $1.607 billion, an increase of 12.3 percent.

CHAPTER ELEVEN

A Strategic Plan Is Developed

THE CHANGES IN THE MARKETPLACE were much on the minds of LabCorp management in 1997. As Tom Mac Mahon saw what was happening in the industry and LabCorp in particular, he decided to be proactive rather than reactive. He and his management team developed a strategic plan to "appropriately address the changing marketplace, including managed care, hospitals, and physician practices." This plan would prove to be a positive step for 1997 and for many years to come.

Mac Mahon said that the Powells had developed a great business model in earlier years. It was perfect for the 1980s and the business atmosphere of that time. However, he said, a change was needed for the remainder of the 1990s and beyond. He said it was essential to "get everyone on the same page" following the merger that had created LabCorp. There had actually been three companies involved in that consolidation. Roche Biomedical Laboratories and National Health Laboratories were the ones actually involved, but NHL had bought Allied Clinical Laboratories immediately prior.

"We needed to be on one strategic plan," he said, citing three factors for such a need.

First, he said, the generation known as the baby boomers was moving into its latter years. As the population grew older, there would be an increasing need for medical testing.

Second, he cited the Center for Molecular Biology that Jim Powell had created in the Research Triangle. That facility offered tremendous opportunities, especially in the newly developed PCR (polymerase chain reaction) method of testing. DNA was a part of it.

PCR was a "profound development," he said. "It changed the entire way we do testing. It was great for all the new genetic testing," such as for HIV testing. "We put a lot of money into it," and "it became the major focus in the lab business," he added. He said that LabCorp people talked about PCR wherever they went to anyone who would listen, and "it catapulted the lab into new ways of testing."

Third, he cited managed care. He said it was recognized that "managed care was here to stay and was going to have a profound effect on testing. Everywhere I talked about older people and managed care and all the new tests" that would be part of the treatment of the older generation.

Mac Mahon said this strategic plan was essential for the company to move ahead in the changing world of the 1990s, stressing LabCorp's place in that shifting environment.

He said it was essential that everyone in the company accept this plan and move ahead together. Mac Mahon told employees at every level, "Everybody has to buy into it [the strategic plan]."

An immediate result of that strategic plan was the formation of new relationships with customers, including contracts with United Health Care Corporation and the Federal Employee Program administered by the Blue Cross and Blue Shield Association.

The company also carried out a number of customer and employee surveys "so we can understand and better serve the expectations and continually improve our high standards of service."

In 1997, core testing was "the heart and soul of LabCorp." Core tests included such routine diagnostic procedures as blood counts, urinalyses, and Pap smears. Every day the company was testing more than 230,000 patient specimens, most of which were core test procedures.

Those tests were done with state-of-the-art automation and sophisticated diagnostic instruments to make certain that each was accomplished with speed and accuracy to benefit the customer.

Transportation of those specimens remained a key part of the entire process. Getting them from the customers to the laboratories and lab results back again continued to be done in the same way as in the early days of Biomedical Reference

Laboratories—by courier, using land and air transportation. By 1997, however, that process that first included a single plane included a fleet of land vehicles and airplanes that logged more than 130 million miles.

By 1997, molecular testing had become such a prominent part of diagnostic testing that in the annual report for that year it was stated, "If core testing is the heart of LabCorp, molecular testing is its spirit.... This specialized area represents the future of diagnostic testing, with its emphasis on unlocking the secrets of DNA sequences and genetic markers. It is here that LabCorp has firmly staked out its position as a leader in creating the clinical laboratory of the future."

By that time, the company's Center for Molecular Biology and Pathology (CMBP) located in North Carolina's Research Triangle Park had become a world-renowned facility by pioneering new applications for polymerase chain reactions.

CMBP was recognized as the most well-established and largest PCR testing facility in the world. It was also staffed by a highly qualified group of MDs and PhDs working exclusively on genetics research and testing.

Using PCR technology, LabCorp increased the accuracy of laboratory testing and "drastically reduced the time it takes to generate results." What had taken weeks now could be done in days, much to the benefit of physicians working to diagnose and treat patients who might be facing life-or-death situations.

A rapidly growing market had developed at that time for companies wanting clinical testing—for new drugs they were trying to bring to market. LabCorp had a relatively small division participating in the clinic trials market, but company management saw the potential for that market and increased its efforts in sales and signing agreements with leading pharmaceutical and biotechnology companies.

More acquisitions in 1998 strengthened the company's position in Florida, Delaware, and Michigan. Also by that time, a partnership had been established with a Belgian company, Virco. That move made LabCorp the first commercial reference laboratory to offer both HIV phenotyping and genotyping—testing that provides physicians with important guidance on which drug therapies to use when treating HIV/AIDS patients.

LabCorp continued as a world leader in the application of PCR technology and its ability to replicate targeted DNA sequences millions of times in a few hours. It was possible at that time to detect a damaged gene or specific disease when only a single cell was affected. More than fifty-five thousand PCR procedures were being done every month, more than at any other clinical laboratory.

LabCorp continued research and development, using DNA for paternity, bone marrow, and forensic testing, as its value was being demonstrated all across the nation, especially in criminal cases. The testing had been developed to the point that matches could be made from the most minute samples—taken, for example, from a strand of hair, a stick of chewing gum, an envelope, or a cigarette butt.

The company also had become a leader in genetic testing. Medical genetics deals with the study of inheritance patterns, particularly those that result in disease. Some inherited diseases are evident at birth, while others become apparent later in life. Biochemical genetics involves the analysis of certain proteins in the blood that are associated with genetic disease.

By 1999 LabCorp had grown to twenty-five major laboratories with approximately nine hundred patient service centers from coast to coast. There were eighteen thousand employees serving more than one hundred thousand physicians, hospitals, managed care organizations, pharmaceutical companies, Fortune 1000 companies, and other clinical laboratories. The company's menu included more than two thousand clinical tests, ranging from simple blood analyses to the world's most sophisticated diagnostic technologies operating at the molecular level.

CHAPTER TWELVE

Centers for Excellence Lead Industry

LABCORP'S CENTERS OF EXCELLENCE were recognized the world over as leaders in the industry. The Center for Molecular Biology and Pathology in the Research Triangle continued to lead in the development and application of polymerase chain reaction technology, a method used to create some of the most sensitive assays ever devised. It was becoming increasingly valuable in diagnostic genetics, oncology, and infectious diseases.

The Center for Occupational Testing had become the world's largest occupational substance abuse testing facility, and the Center for Esoteric Testing located in the Powell Laboratory Complex in Burlington performed the largest volume of rare analyses in the network.

The year 2000 was an extremely good year for LabCorp. In fact, "It was unquestionably the best year ever for our company," according to Chairman and Chief Executive Officer Thomas P. Mac Mahon in the 2000 annual report to shareholders. It was a year "when the company consistently exceeded expectations."

New contracts were made with CIGNA HealthCare, Aetna, and United Healthcare, the three largest national managed-care companies. Agreements with the Health Trust Purchasing Group and AmeriNet brought contact with many new hospitals, surgery centers, clinics, and physicians.

Several laboratories were acquired during the year, the largest of which was National Genetics Institute (NGI) in Los Angeles. That acquisition improved the company's position in genomic testing. It also allowed the company to gain NGI's ultra-sensitive hepatitis C testing capability.

Also acquired were the San Diego based POISONLAB Inc.'s occupational substance abuse and clinical toxicology testing business; certain clinical testing assets of Bio-Diagnostics Laboratories in Torrance, California; and Pathology Medical Laboratories in San Diego.

By 2001, genomics had grown to major importance in the laboratory testing industry. In fact, almost all the annual report that year was devoted to genomics, because, as Mac Mahon said, "By far, the most important growth story for LabCorp is the evolving dynamic between laboratory testing and genomics. Simply put: the most compelling growth is in the science itself."

The genome is the entire DNA content that is present within one cell of an organism, and genomics is an area within genetics that concerns the sequencing and analysis of an organism's genome.

The 2001 annual report stated,

> The evolving science of genomics is a revolution creating the most profound opportunities for improved medical care in more than a century. The benefits of being diagnosed earlier, more effective medicines, and better treatment programs that will derive from the mapping of the human genome are nearly beyond measure. LabCorp stands to be an early beneficiary of this new era.

The report examined a number of things essential to the company if it were to gain the maximum benefit from that revolution—scientific credentials, innovation, alliances and partnerships, acquisitions and clinical trials. In 2001 LabCorp was at the cutting edge in every one of those categories.

In 2001 Viro-Med Laboratories became a part of LabCorp, bringing into the company's list of technologies one of the leading laboratories in molecular microbial testing using real-time PCR platforms. ViroMed was a Minneapolis company and a national leader in specialized disease testing.

In the same year, the company acquired Path Lab in New England, adding thirty-five patient service centers in that part of the country.

On September 11, 2001, Karen McFadden drove to Raleigh-Durham International Airport from Burlington to pick up some clients who were coming to meet with LabCorp management. That was the day, of course, of the terrorist attacks on the World Trade Center in New York City and elsewhere—9/11, as we have come to remember it. One of her passengers was from New York City, and it was a stressful situation, to say the least.

McFadden remembers that LabCorp management immediately looked for a way to help victims of the attack as well as their families. Tom Mac Mahon and others on the management team decided to open all LabCorp facilities across the nation to relatives of victims. Blood samples could be taken and sent to the New York City Department of Health, and they could be used in DNA testing to determine the identity of many of the victims. McFadden remembers that the company did this without any charge to anyone. It was a matter of, "What can we do?"

All airplanes had been grounded, so everything had to be moved by automobile, but it worked out. McFadden said that other labs—major competitors—joined in the effort and worked together to get the job done.

She had lived in a small town in New Jersey previously, and eleven victims were from that town, some of whom she knew. Friends called her for help, and she was able to assist several in getting it. She also remembered one particular problem among all the chaos of that day. One individual involved in all the testing that day had "Blood" as a last name. That name became confused with the tests, but the issue was finally resolved.

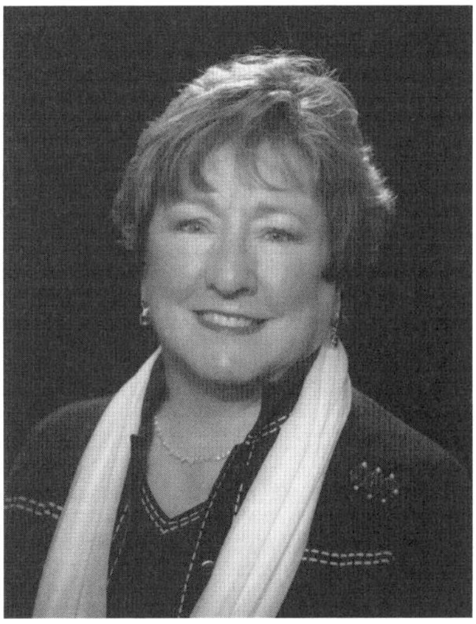
Karen McFadden

McFadden was another longtime member of the LabCorp family, having joined Roche Clinical Reference Laboratory in 1974 in Raritan, New Jersey. She had studied to be a lab technician and was in a hospital lab, where her job was "the lowest on the totem pole." Then a recruiter from Roche contacted her. She said Roche had a great reputation, "so I thought maybe I will go work for them." She did just that, joining Roche in January 1974. She worked first in hematology and then in blood banking.

She was a New Jersey girl from a small town where "everyone was either Italian or Irish and either Catholic or Protestant," and she said it was quite a culture shock when she went to the Roche facility. People working there were from a variety of nationalities and religions.

"It looked like the United Nations," she said. There were people there from China, Pakistan, Indonesia, Panama, and other locations, and they all had their own food and their own languages.

Early in her work there, the company was growing rapidly. Sometimes they had so much work coming in that they could not get it out. The lab was in operation twenty-four hours a day, and some of the employees would occasionally stay in hotels nearby in order to save travel time.

"Everybody learned from that situation," she said.

McFadden said she began to notice that the sales representatives did not always know much about testing, so she decided to see if she could get into that side of the operation and lend her lab experience to sales. In the late 1970s she became a sales representative in New Jersey. Later her territory expanded to include Connecticut and parts of New York.

"I was pretty successful," she said, working with large accounts, including hospitals, nursing homes, and even jails. Her success led her to the position of sales manager for the area from the Bronx to Maine and then sales officer for the Northeast. At that point, the entire northeastern area was run by women.

"That was unheard of at the time," she said, and for three successive years, the national YWCA presented its Twin Award, highlighting women in industry, to the LabCorp family. In 1991 the award was won by Pat Frele, by McFadden in 1992, and by the company itself in 1993.

When the company merged with National Health, McFadden said, "I dealt with all the health plans," and then later, "I was asked to come to headquarters to head the managed care part" of the business. She dealt with all the major health plan companies across the nation. In that position she worked with contracts, relationships, and other issues relating to managed care and insurance. She was still in that position in 2016, forty-two years after joining Roche, and was located in Burlington.

Dynacare became a part of the company in 2002, bringing with it locations in twenty-one states and Canada, broadening LabCorp's footprint, and enhancing service to clients and their patients by having more conveniently located patient service centers and on-site testing facilities.

Another agreement, this one with Myriad Genetics, made it possible for physicians to send patients to one of LabCorp's patient service centers for Myriad Genetics' predisposition test for the BRCA mutation associated with breast cancer. This testing, combined with LabCorp's extensive menu of other genetic tests, improved the ability of physicians to more quickly answer the questions of their patients who were facing critical issues. Expectant mothers were able to learn if they were one of the more than 10 million who carried the genetic mutations known to cause cystic fibrosis, allowing them to make more informed decisions about family planning. Patients were able to learn more quickly if they had colorectal cancer, and if so, how aggressive that cancer might be. Early testing for that and other cancers improved the chances for their elimination, and when that occurred, testing would confirm if the patient was cancer-free.

As new tests continued to be developed, physicians' and patients' questions could be more readily and accurately answered. Other agreements and collaborations continued to widen the scope of services offered by LabCorp and made it more convenient for physicians and patients to receive testing in an always quick and efficient manner.

DIANON was a company that was known for its capabilities in specific organ systems and clinical disciplines of uropathology, dermatopathology, and gastrointestinal pathology. That company became part of LabCorp in 2003.

All these moves continued to serve LabCorp's goal of building the strongest anatomic pathology capabilities in the world.

In 2003 Chairman and CEO Tom Mac Mahon said,

> Six years ago LabCorp embarked on a journey guided by a strategic plan. Today this plan remains more relevant than ever. Like a well-drawn roadmap, clear planning is essential to securing success in life, and in business as well. LabCorp's substantial accomplishments in 2003—in financial performance, in scientific leadership, in service to patients and providers—were the result of knowing exactly where we

> wanted to go and which roads to take. Indeed, our success and growth to date all relate directly to the execution of the strategic plan we first devised six years ago.

That plan was to make LabCorp the leader in the industry in achieving long-term growth and profitability by strengthening its nationwide core testing business and expanding its higher-growth, higher-value esoteric and genomic businesses.

As a result, Mac Mahon said, "LabCorp today has become one of the largest clinical laboratory organizations in the world as well as the leader in developing and commercializing a broad menu of sophisticated assays that provide critical information to physicians and their patients."

By that point, LabCorp had more than eleven hundred patient service centers and thirty-one testing laboratories serving patients in all fifty states. More than 340,000 specimens were processed daily for more than 240,000 customers.

LabCorp continued its strong growth in 2004. In fact, its revenues exceeded $3 billion for the first time, with net earnings of $363 million.

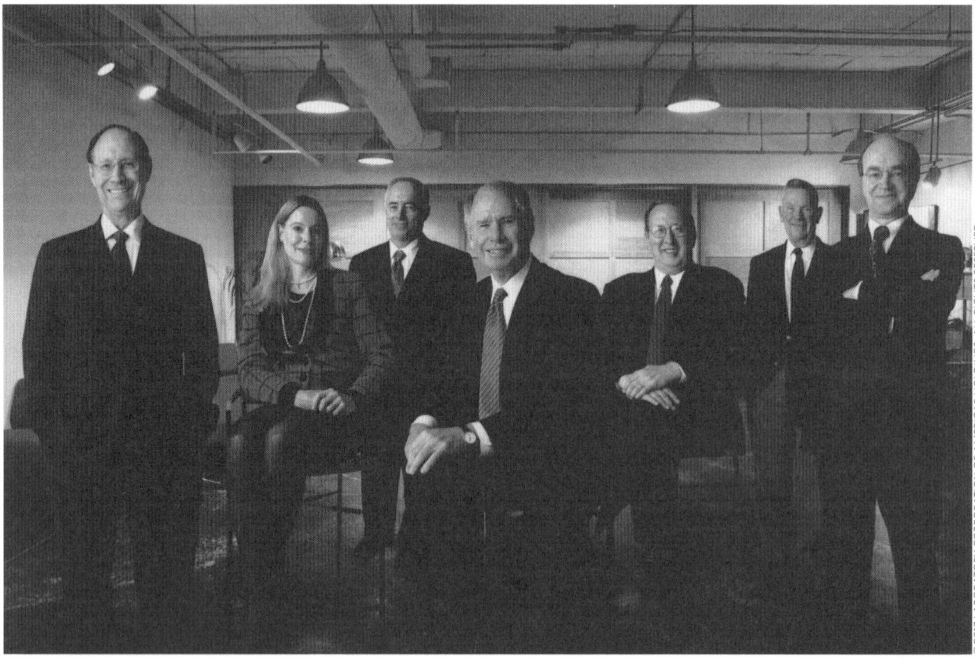

The LabCorp board of directors in 2004, left to right, Arthur N. Rubenstein, Wendy E. Lane, Robert E. Mittlestaedt Jr., Chairman and CEO Thomas Mac Mahon, M. Keith Weikel, Andrew G. Wallace, Jean-Luc Bélingard

These achievements were not overlooked by others in the business world. In fact, Standard and Poor's recognized the company's growth, financial strength, and industry position by adding LabCorp to the S&P 500 Index—one of the most widely used and recognized benchmarks of US equity performance.

By 2005 laboratory testing accounted for only 4 percent of the cost of health care in the nation. However, that testing influenced as much as 80 percent of all subsequent health-care decisions and costs.

As the population grew older, health-care costs would continue to rise, and LabCorp management felt the company could help make sure the money was spent on treatment and therapies that most benefitted the patients. Testing's role became even more important, especially in the area of cancer, where occurrence dramatically increases with age. LabCorp was already a leader in oncology testing, putting the company in a place of leadership as health care for the older individual became more and more important.

CHAPTER THIRTEEN

The Focus Is on Cancer

LABCORP CONTINUED TO FOCUS on cancer testing as more than a million Americans were diagnosed with some form of cancer each year. Clinical testing saved lives through prevention, detection, treatment, and monitoring of cancer. A good example of that fact was in cervical cancer testing. Pap screening technology reduced the rate of cervical cancer in dramatic fashion over the years, and then came the AutoCyte (TriPath) Imaging System that originated at RBL and improved things even more. LabCorp also uses the CYTYC thin-layer and imaging system.

LabCorp was the first national laboratory to offer thin-layer and image-guided Pap testing services. As a result, demand for image-guided testing increased dramatically—from almost zero at the end of 2004 to an annualized rate of 2.3 million tests at the end of 2005.

Advances continued as well in other areas of testing, including a pharmacogenetic test to help physicians better prescribe medications. This testing allowed doctors not only to prescribe more effective medications and save costs but also to avoid giving a medication that might cause serious drug interactions.

During 2005 the company acquired US LABS and Esoterix at a total investment of $306 million. US LABS strengthened the company's position in cancer diagnostics, and Esoterix brought other new tests to the LabCorp menu.

In 2007, in what company officials called a historic move, LabCorp entered into a ten-year agreement with UnitedHealthCare that made LabCorp its exclusive national laboratory. This allowed UnitedHealthCare to offer a comprehensive suite of services to its members all across the United States. To meet the new demand, LabCorp needed to expand its facilities, so more than four hundred new patient service centers were opened and twelve hundred new employees were added to make certain that customers continued to receive the highest level of service. Company officials called this a "landmark contract." "In fact," it was stated, "we believe there is no other relationship in the lab industry of such scope, scale, or timeframe."

This was the largest such relationship, but in years that followed, a number of other expanded relationships were made with managed care companies. In order to achieve such relationships, company spokespersons said three things were essential—quality, innovation, and convenience—three qualities the company had continually stressed.

During 2006 Thomas Mac Mahon retired as president and chief executive officer but remained as chairman of the board. David P. King became chief executive officer, having previously served as executive vice president and chief operating officer.

King was in private practice for seventeen years and a law partner with Hogan & Hartson L.L.P. in Baltimore when he was first introduced to LabCorp. He worked with the company on the government investigation that went on during the mid-1990s, collaborating closely with Jim Powell and Brad Smith. That issue was settled in 1996, but King still did some private litigation for the company. He also filled in for the compliance officer for a period of time. The District of Columbia native is the son of a college professor who taught at the University of Illinois and at Berkeley in California. King graduated high school in Berkeley, then received his bachelor's degree from Princeton University and his JD from the University of Pennsylvania.

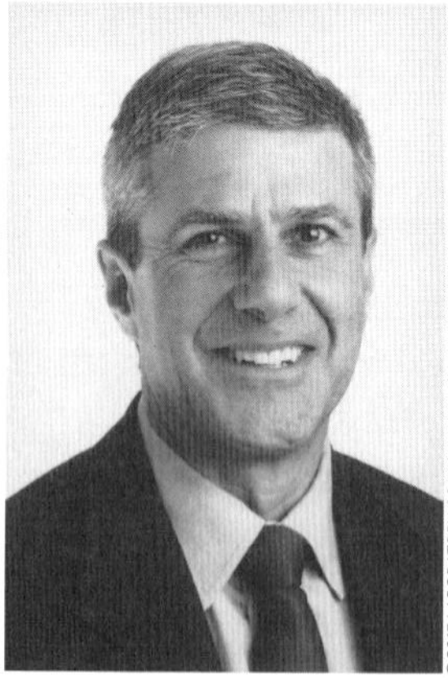

David P. King

For about three and a half years he was an assistant US attorney in the Justice Department. While at Hogan and Hartson, John Roberts, now Chief Justice of the US Supreme Court, was also with the firm.

King made many friends in the LabCorp organization during his work on the government issue. "I liked the people a lot," he said. There were discussions about him coming to LabCorp, but initially he decided to remain in law practice.

But then King married and had a family, and as time passed, he said the demands of his law practice caused him to spend too much time away from his family. So in September 2001 he became senior vice president, general counsel, and chief compliance officer for LabCorp.

In January 2004 he became executive vice president of strategic planning and corporate development, and then he rose to executive vice president and chief operating officer in December 2005. On January 1, 2007, he became president, CEO, and a board member.

The acquisitions continued in 2006 when LabCorp bought Litholink Corporation. Litholink provided assistance for physicians and their patients with outcomes management. The impact of those outcomes management programs in preventing the recurrence of disease or the progression of disease was quite impressive.

Also at that time more than forty new tests were introduced in areas such as oncology, infectious disease, immunology, genetics, coagulation, and women's health. In doing so, the company continued its plan of following two common themes in such introductions: targeting areas where the market was not meeting a clear need and utilizing new technology that was increasingly oriented toward the goal of becoming the leading laboratory in personalized medicine.

LabCorp made expansions in New York, Chicago, and St. Louis. The acquisition of Diagnostic Services Inc. Laboratories in western Florida added new labs in a heavily populated area, and the addition of PA Labs, Inc. in Muncie, Indiana, just outside Indianapolis, provided exposure in the twelfth-largest metropolitan area in the nation. Those deals closed in 2007.

In 2007 Jean Neff decided it was time to retire. Jean was senior vice president of operations and had a career with the company dating back to 1978.

As she came to retirement, she said, "It is overwhelming when you look back. The commitment of a core group of people [in this company] was phenomenal. We did what we had to do," she said, repeating a phrase heard over and over from many others who were a part of the family of LabCorp and its predecessors over the years.

Jean got her start in a small laboratory operated by a doctor in Anderson, South Carolina. She was a medical technician there. She knew Paul Hoffner, a vice president with Biomedical Laboratories in Burlington, and she knew the company as it was her

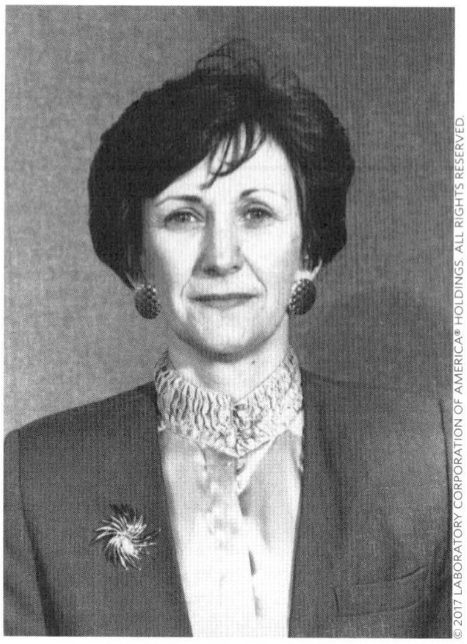

Jean Neff

little lab's major competition. She decided to call Paul Hoffner and see if she could get a job with Biomedical instead of constantly competing with them. She called Hoffner and asked for a job. He told her, "Come up and meet with me." She did just that, going to the Rainey Street facility, as York Court was still under construction at the time.

"Paul wanted me to work with the sales representatives and resolve problems with the customers," she said. The sales representatives were taking so much time dealing with customer problems that it was affecting their sales. She said Jim Powell was not warm to the idea of such a job, however. He said there was not enough demand for such a job and the company could not afford it.

Neff told him to give her ninety days, and she became a technical sales representative focusing on customer problems, not sales. She passed the ninety-day mark and never looked back. In that job, she might go into a hospital and work with management in solving problems relating to testing done through her company or help other customers deal with their issues.

"I did that five or six years and ran all over the country," and she said her work boosted sales as well. After chasing around the country all that time, she began to tire of the travel.

"I went to [financial officer] Haywood Cochrane and told him the travel was wearing me down," adding that she needed a change, maybe into sales or sales support.

Cochrane told her, "We don't know what you do, but you do it well," and he said he would keep her request in mind.

For a while she worked with one of the company's facilities in the Washington, DC, area, and then she received a call from Burlington. A general manager was needed in the laboratory there to work in customer service. Neff said she did that for several years, working inside the company for the first time. Then she took over the paternity testing laboratory, which was then operated as a separate entity within the company. She became an assistant vice president at that point. She later became senior vice president for operations for the Northeast Division, working in New Jersey for seven years.

"Those were my best years," she said, noting that she had $300 million in business in that division. She was there when LabCorp was formed, and at that time she came back to Burlington and ran sales for the Carolinas as senior vice president for operations.

Jean Neff was like so many other members of the LabCorp organization who started as lab technicians or in other spots, some making minimum wage, but who rose through the company, contributing to its growth while assuming positions of increasing importance.

A Three-Year Plan

The company announced a three-year plan in 2007: "LabCorp 2010." The long-standing commitment to running the best lab in the nation was the reason for the plan, which would provide new and improved tools to its employees, increase automation in the preanalytical process, make use of robotics in the laboratory, optimize logistics, and maximize the supply chain.

"Personalized medicine" was a term that had the full attention of LabCorp scientists by 2008. The term emerged after the company opened the Center for Molecular Biology and Pathology in the Research Triangle in 1990, and the company had worked hard since that time to further develop it. A quote in the 2008 annual report said this:

> If no two of us are alike, then let's treat each patient differently. This simple logic is the basis of a new era of health care that is rapidly evolving.
>
> Scientific advances of the molecular and genetic level are making the concept of personalized medicine a reality—today. This new era means new opportunities and new growth.
>
> LabCorp is staking a leadership claim as the clinical laboratory for personalized medicine. We are in an excellent position....

President and CEO King added that "LabCorp intends to continue to lead the laboratory industry in the movement toward personalized medicine. We expect this area to be a key driver of growth for the company going forward. We are in an excellent position to realize this goal."

The year 2008 brought an economic downturn of significant proportions, but LabCorp enjoyed a solid year with a 10.7 percent increase in sales to $4.5 billion.

The purchase of Tandem Laboratories in 2008 and Monogram Biosciences in 2009

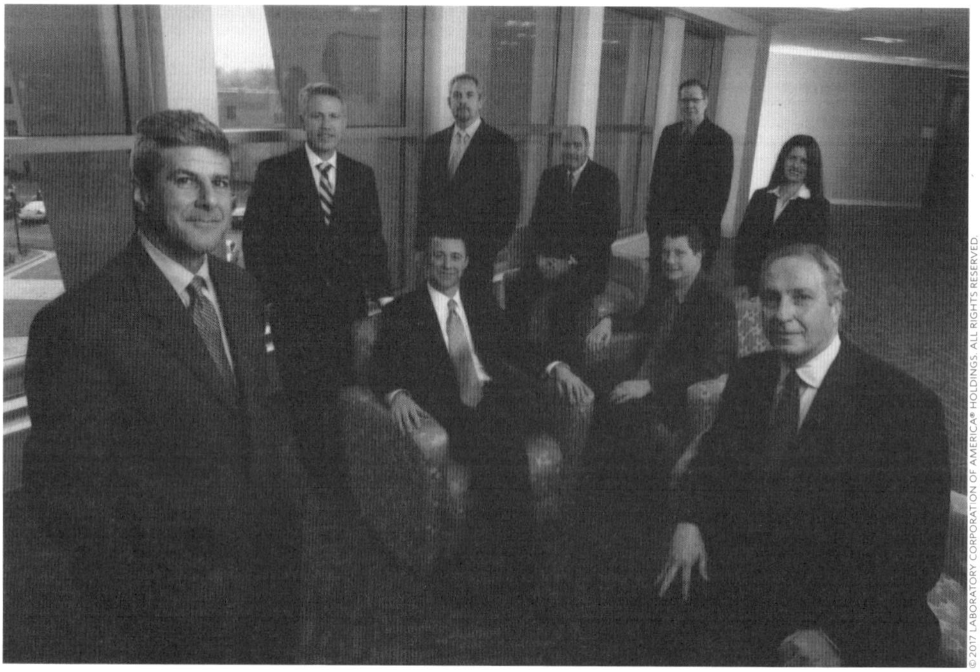

2008 management team with president and CEO Dave King at left, continuing left to right, Scott Walton, Brad Hayes, Andrew Conrad, Jay Boyle, Bill Bonello, Sam Eberts, Lidia Fonesca, Don Hardison

opened still more doors. Tandem was a leader in bioanalytical and immunoanalytical contract research. Their research supported pharmaceutical and biotechnology companies with their discovery, preclinical, and clinical drug programs. Monogram was a recognized leader in the discovery and commercialization of products in the treatment of HIV, cancer, and other serious diseases. Monogram brought with it a state-of-the-art complex molecular assay called Trofile. It identifies the cell type of every individual patient's HIV and was the standard in its diagnosis area.

In October 2008 LabCorp opened its new corporate headquarters on Spring Street in downtown Burlington. Dedication took place on December 11.

The structure contained 115,000 square feet and represented an investment of $12 million, with another $8 million in furniture and computers. Approximately 150 employees moved into the building, coming from the 1937-era Federal Building just across the Spring Street–Maple Avenue intersection, from the former First Federal Savings and Loan Building on Davis Street, and seventeen other downtown locations. The new building houses management, human resources, and the sales and

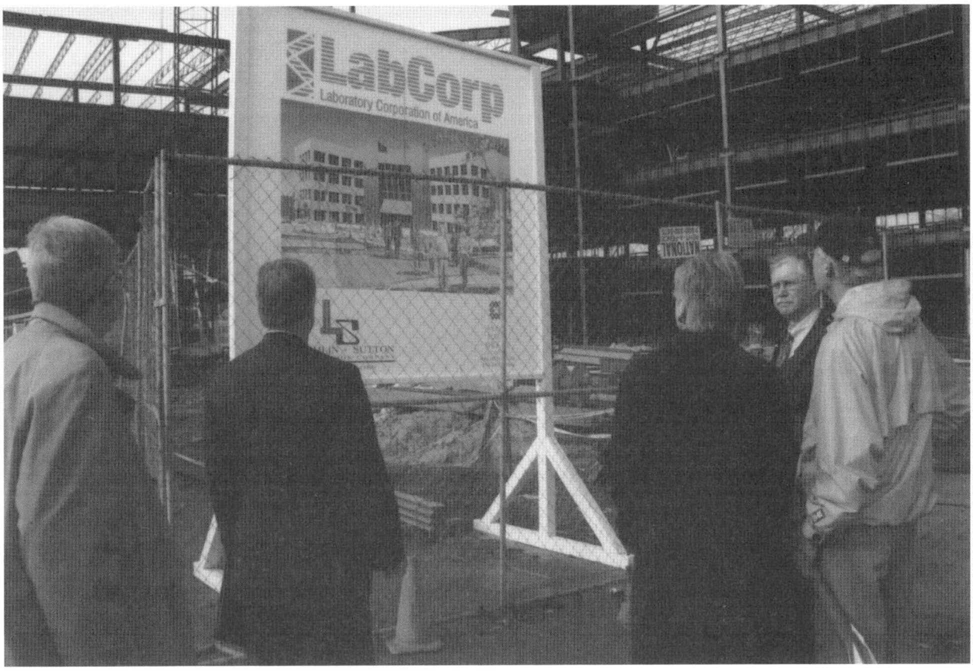

Company officials tour new national headquarters building in construction

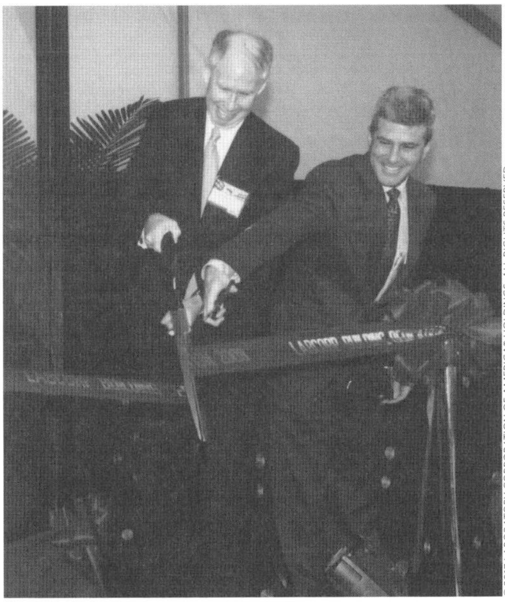

Tom Mac Mahon and Dave King cut the ribbon for new headquarters site in 2008

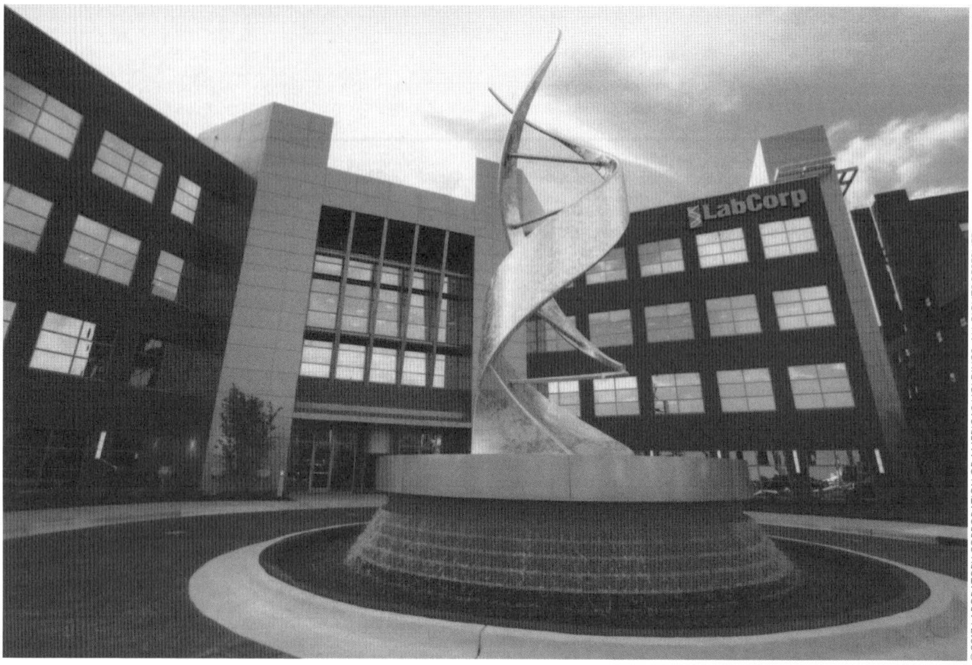

The double helix stands in front of new headquarters building

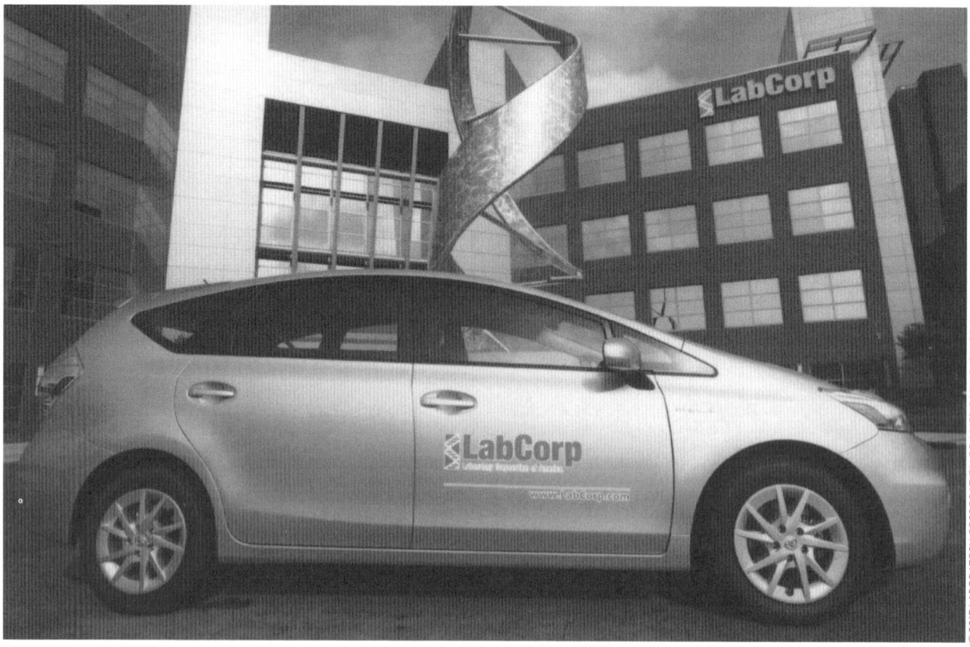

LabCorp enters a new era in facilities—a new headquarters building—and in logistics—modern vehicles

marketing departments. Some of the vacated sites would later be given to local nonprofit organizations.

A thirty-six-foot stainless steel sculpture of a double helix—a symbol of the company—was erected in front of the building in May while construction was still going on. The new headquarters facility was dedicated to Thomas Mac Mahon who had just retired as CEO. He was honored for his "leadership and service that helped transform LabCorp and the entire lab industry."

The paint on the new headquarters was hardly dry before LabCorp had approval from the city of Burlington for a new office building in West Burlington. Burlington's city council at its December 2008 meeting rezoned 22.96 acres for office and institutional use. The company said there were no specific plans for the property, but an office building would likely go there.

Along about this time, Lew Annucci was traveling the country as a corporate trainer in billing. Lew said he was "caught up in the conversion team" after the formation of LabCorp in the 1990s, and he traveled until about 2008.

Annucci was one of the employees who had begun his career with the Kings County Research Laboratory in Brooklyn, New York. He said he was hired in 1968 in a lab that had 150 to 200 people. "It was a small lab, but we did a lot of testing." His first job was as a lab assistant, and his duties included tasks like washing the glassware used in the lab.

Today a potential employee might have to undergo a long interview and testing process of several days or even weeks, but Annucci had a much simpler route to his job. On his twentieth birthday, September 16, 1968, he applied for a job at KCRL. That night he went to work on the third shift.

KCRL moved from the Brooklyn lab to a lab in West Caldwell, New Jersey, and then it was not long until KCRL became a part of Roche Clinical Labs' diagnostic division. At that point, everything moved to Raritan, New Jersey. Dr. Herbert Kuppermann operated KCRL and built a national reputation in endocrinology.

Like many others, Annucci moved up through various positions during his forty-five years of service. He went from washing lab bottles to tech support to distribution services to accounting to billing. He saw the company grow from its beginning, and he saw a lot of the company locations, traveling all over the country. He was in Burlington in April 2016 for the retirement of a friend, and he said, "I must have been in Burlington three hundred times, but this is the first time I drove [from New Jersey]. I always flew before [on company business]."

In March 2009 an article in the *Burlington Times-News* revealed plans for LabCorp and Duke University to operate and manage a new biorepository facility.

The facility was planned for the North Carolina Research Facility in Kannapolis, North Carolina, and would store human biological samples for a wide variety of customers such as academic centers, research organizations, and health-care providers. Plans were for the facility to house up to 10 million samples. David P. King, LabCorp CEO, said, "The combined capabilities of our organizations through the biorepository will further our leadership in personalized medicine and will lead to new discoveries and new diagnostic biomarkers and will expand the services it offers commercial clients."

In May 2008 King became board chairman and CEO as former board chair Thomas Mac Mahon continued as a board member.

At the end of the first decade of the twenty-first century, LabCorp was the second-largest clinical laboratory in the nation. Its 2010 revenue was $5 billion. More than 270 million tests were being performed annually for 220,000 clients, and there were over seventeen hundred patient service centers and fifty-one primary laboratories.

The company had eight specialized Centers of Excellence, eight thousand patient service technicians/phlebotomists, and twenty-seven hundred service representatives/couriers. Eight aircraft were operating.

CHAPTER FOURTEEN

The Expansion Continues

IN 2010 LABCORP GREATLY EXPANDED its capabilities in genetics and oncology services with the acquisition of Genzyme Genetics, a business unit of the Genzyme Corporation.

In that acquisition, LabCorp obtained a license to use the Genzyme Genetics name for about one year. A new name would be introduced in 2012, and in the ensuing months, LabCorp executives worked to connect the services of that company into LabCorp so as to better serve clients. There was also work in the area of joining the oncology capabilities of US LABS and Genzyme Genetics into a single offering.

In 2012, it was announced that the brand name would be Integrated Genetics for the reproductive portion of the Genzyme Genetics business, and the US LABS and Genzyme Genetics oncology would operate under the brand name Integrated Oncology.

LabCorp obtained Orchid Cellmark in December 2011. This acquisition expanded LabCorp's presence on the international stage, as the company had DNA testing facilities in the United States and the United Kingdom.

In April 2012 LabCorp announced a new global name, CellMark Forensics, in recognition of many years of company service to law enforcement and legal communities in the United States and the world. The new name combined two well established brands—LabCorp Forensic Identity and Orchid CellMark. Cellmark Forensics is LabCorp's fully accredited resource, focused exclusively on the company's market-leading testing expertise in DNA.

On July 31, 2012, MEDTOX Scientific Inc. became a part of LabCorp. This was another specialized testing company, adding to the company's position in specialized toxicology and medical drug monitoring testing services.

In 2012 also, the company debuted its LabCorp Beacon platform, described in its annual report as an end-to-end solution that provided significant value to all healthcare stakeholders.

LabCorp Beacon: Analytics provided business-intelligence tools to hospitals, physician practices, and accountable care organizations. Beacon's assets and functionalities included physician, patient, and payer portals; electronic ordering; enhanced reports; lab analyses that provided trending of patient, test, and population data; and clinical support tools. Those intelligent tools helped customers better manage productivity and patient outcome metrics. LabCorp maintained more than six hundred clinical quality measures.

LabCorp Beacon: Patient allowed patients to take control of their health information: receiving and sharing lab results, making lab appointments, paying bills, and setting up automatic alerts and notifications for the whole family.

Weather became a factor in the company's operations in October 2012. Hurricane Sandy, one of the worst storms to ever hit the United States, roared up the Eastern Seaboard and caused damage the likes of which had never been recorded in areas of New Jersey and Maryland and then into New York and New England. That storm had a devastating impact on all business activity for several months.

The Mac Mahon Era Ends

Also in October of 2012 it was announced that Thomas Mac Mahon would step down as a member of the board at the end of his term on May 8, 2013. He had been a director since 1995 and was the company's president and CEO from 1997 until he retired from those duties in 2006. From 2007 to 2009 he served as nonexecutive chairman of the board.

Although he retired from his LabCorp duties, he continued to be active in the business community. He later served as lead director of the Express Scripts board of directors and a member of the boards of PharMerica Corporation, SynapDx Corporation, Aushon BioSystems, and Ortho Clinical Diagnostics.

He is also an executive partner of the venture capital group Flare Capital Partners.

In 2004 he was recognized by *Forbes* magazine, and again in 2010 by the Harvard Business Review, as one of the one hundred best-performing CEOs in the world.

He is a trustee emeritus of Elon University and in 2015 was chairman of the board of trustees of Saint Peter's University.

In an interview some years after his retirement from LabCorp, he continued to express his passion for the future work to be done by the company. "I have great hope" for LabCorp, he said. "We have the ability now to test anything."

He was particularly interested in the testing of drugs, making sure they are investigated rigidly to determine if they are effective and will do the job they are intended to do. He said the acquisition of Covance (in 2015), a drug development services company, would be a major step forward in that process.

Mac Mahon said, "Everybody is different," and they tolerate a drug differently, "and we need to understand how it works in our body." He said his "dream of personalized medicine" will lead to better diagnosis and treatment for every patient.

Mac Mahon praised the vision of Jim Powell in the 1960s when he opened his laboratory in Burlington. "It has had a profound impact," he said and "has affected people around the world." He called LabCorp a "wonderful company."

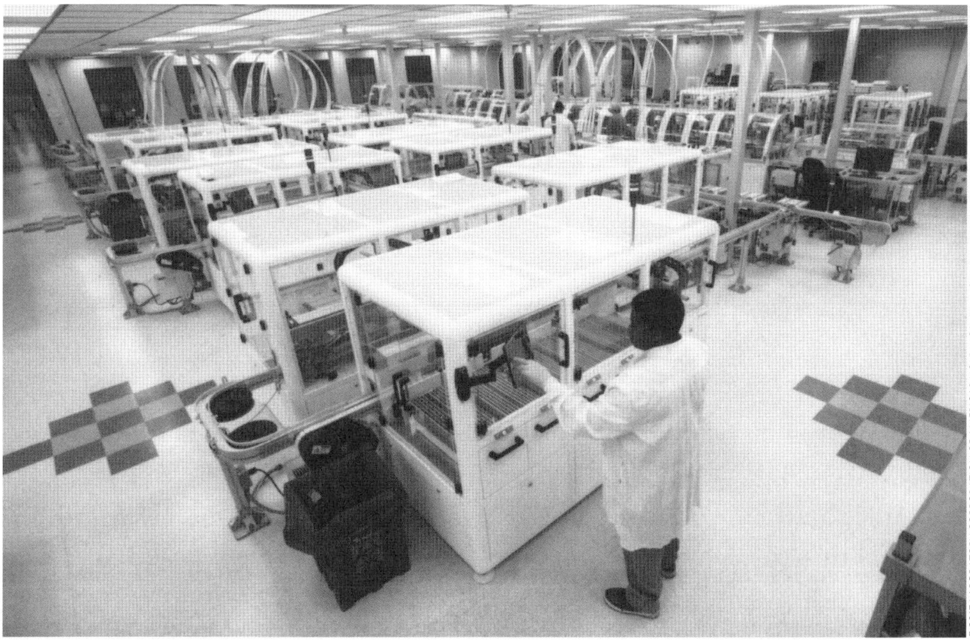

LabCorp facilities are among the most modern in the world

Almost from the beginning of Biomedical Laboratories in 1969, the company had used aircraft as a major part of its operations. The planes ferried medical samples to be tested from distant points to the lab to help speed up the process and get results back to physicians and hospitals at the earliest possible moment. Patient lives often depended on that speed.

Over the years there were some minor incidents involving LabCorp planes, but there had been nothing serious until January 16, 2013.

On that morning, pilot David Gamble was the only person aboard the single-engine Pilatus PC-12 as it took off from the Burlington-Alamance Regional Airport. Gamble was on a trip to deliver interoffice mail to New Jersey and was bound for the Morristown, New Jersey, airport.

The plane was in the air only four minutes before it crashed and exploded in a vacant field in north Burlington. Gamble was killed instantly.

He crashed near a heavily populated area, yet Gamble managed to avoid hitting aparment buildings nearby. In a show of respect for Gamble, hundreds of his co-workers and many senior executives at LabCorp attended his funeral.

LabCorp continued its emphasis on scientific vision and leadership in 2014 when it added another 174-test menu and automation enhancements. The company continued its focus on expansion of existing programs in molecular diagnostics as well as the introduction of new assay and assay platforms through licensing partnerships, acquisitions, and internal developments.

New tests were added in many areas, including cardiovascular disease risk assessment, infectious diseases, breast cancer tests, coagulation, obstetrics and gynecology, and genomics.

The company also launched a new business in 2014 through its Enlighten Health initiative, which provided tools and services for patients and health-care providers. Enlighten Health Genomics was started "to offer state-of-the-art diagnostic capabilities, NGS analysis, and interpretation and informed genetic counseling" using a team of "accomplished geneticists."

In an article in the *Burlington Times-News,* David P. King, chairman and CEO, said, "Enlighten Health Genomics is an important part of LabCorp's strategy to capitalize on the unique assets, create new sources of revenue from our core capabilities, and meaningfully differentiate us from competitors. The launch of this business is another tangible step in the development of Enlighten Health, our initiative to create innovative tools and capabilities to enhance patient care," he said.

Duke University genetics professor David Goldstein, now at Columbia Presbyterian, who was selected as chairman of the Enlighten Health Genomics' Scientific Advisory Board, said patients with serious genetic conditions will require a thorough interpretation of their genome.

"Our goal is to offer innovative and affordable diagnostic solutions to broad populations, making genomics a routine part of clinical decisions," he said.

LabCorp's position in DNA testing was enhanced in late 2014 with the acquisition of Bode Technology Group.

Bode was a DNA testing company and was acquired from SolutionPoint International. Bode and its division Chromosomal Labs provided specialized forensic DNA analysis and other services to the international market. With the acquisition it joined with LabCorp's US- and UK-based DNA Identity and Cellmark Forensics businesses. Bode would be working with federal and state government law enforcement agencies and crime labs.

Also in 2014, the company announced that it had begun allergy testing through Thermo Fisher Scientific. The agreement between the two companies gave LabCorp access to Thermo Fisher's "unmatched allergy testing portfolio of more than 600 allergens and 100 allergen components." Dr. Mark Brecher, LabCorp's chief medical officer, said this was an important expansion, allowing the company "to provide innovative testing technologies that facilitate earlier and more accurate diagnosis, treatment, and monitoring of diseases and medical conditions."

The company estimated that some 60 million people in the country were affected by allergies, and the agreement with Thermo Fisher would greatly enhance the ability to deal with the problem.

LabCorp announced in March 2014 that Glenn A. Eisenberg had been named executive vice president and chief financial officer, replacing Brad Hayes. Eisenberg had most recently been chief financial officer for the Timken Co., a leading global manufacturer of highly engineered bearings and other steels and related products and services. Hayes retired after a seventeen-year career as LabCorp's CFO.

In April 2014 the Burlington Times-News reported that LabCorp would be moving 975 employees—nearly half of its downtown employees—to a facility in Guilford County, vacating five older buildings in need of renovation in downtown Burlington. Employees were to be moved to a former call center off Interstate 85-40 near McLeansville in Guilford County, some twenty miles west of Burlington. No jobs were being eliminated. In all, LabCorp had fifteen buildings in downtown Burlington.

LabCorp officials said that more than 2,500 employees would remain in Alamance County after the relocation, including 200 in its headquarters. Plans were being made at that time to add another 140 employees at the Powell Building on the York Court campus, home to the company's largest US lab.

David King said the decision "was not without sleepless nights and cost in the way the city sees us." He said it was a most difficult decision to make, as it greatly affected the community in which much of the company's history was located.

Two years after that move was made, LabCorp donated three of the buildings it had vacated to Impact Alamance, an umbrella organization under which a number of nonprofits in Burlington and Alamance operate. Impact Alamance is a wing of Cone Health and distributes some $2 million annually to nonprofits involved in the health, educational, and economic sectors of the community. The buildings included some of the most historic in downtown Burlington, one of which is on the National Register of Historic Places.

Covance: A Major Acquisition

On November 2, 2014, LabCorp acquired Covance, a company based in Princeton, New Jersey, and described as a "comprehensive drug development services company and a leader in nutritional analysis." Covance brought its 12,500 employees in sixty countries into the merged company, making LabCorp an operation with more than 45,500 employees and annual net revenues greater than $8.3 billion. With this move, LabCorp became the world's leading health-care diagnostics company, and it also took a major position in the world's drug development business.

Covance dealt in innovative drug development solutions, "generating more safety and efficacy data to support drug approvals than any other company in the world," according to a company press release. Covance was the market leader in central laboratory, bioanalysis, and toxicology services, and a leading provider of clinical trial solutions. The press release also said, "By providing comprehensive clinical laboratory services and end-to-end support solutions, the LabCorp-Covance union will provide resources for clients and, ultimately, the lives of the patients they serve."

Denise McFadden was happy in her role at Covance at the time, having served in several capacities with the company that was a leader in clinical testing. She said she was quite surprised when she got a call one morning from her sister Karen, a long-time employee of LabCorp, telling her, "You have been bought by LabCorp."

McFadden was shocked to say the least, as she had been with LabCorp in earlier years but had quit. She was selling HIV testing to pharmaceutical companies at the time. Her story is one that has extended over a number of years and has been part of the evolution of the company from its early days.

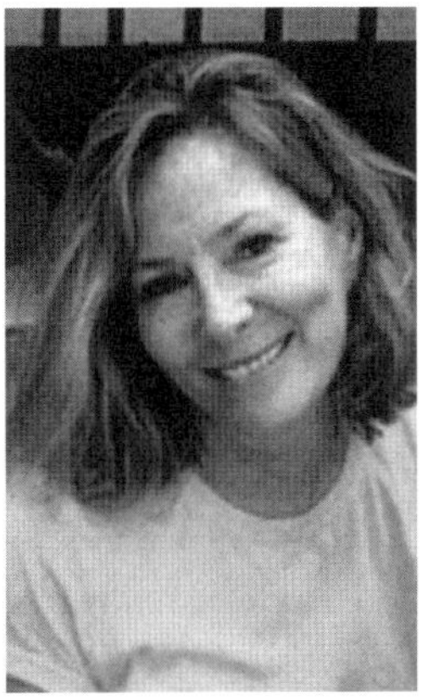

Denise McFadden

After Denise McFadden left LabCorp, she took off for a year and traveled the world, becoming involved in work with an orphanage in Tanzania. "I wanted to do more at the time, so I decided to go back to work and make money so I could go back" to Tanzania.

A friend led her to an interview with Covance, and after meeting with them nineteen times, she joined them as a sales representative. Today she is senior business development director with the Covance Division in Indianapolis, Indiana.

She first joined Roche Clinical Laboratories in Raritan, New Jersey, in 1976 in customer service. "There were only five of us. We called lab results to the offices" of doctors. A year later she moved into data entry as a keypunch operator.

In those early days, "samples came in and we actually handled them—with no gloves." Information from the cards that came with the samples was punched into the computer, and the testing process was completed.

Later Denise went back to computer services, where an issue had developed "when the key computer person left with a lot of stuff" necessary to operations. She said she helped as she could in an effort to resolve the problems that had arisen.

Later she was bothered by a problem in her department. She said customer service workers often had to leave their patient calls to go in and out of the labs for information. She started the Customer Service Technical Department to correct that.

"We were runners for customer service, and I ran that for a long time," she said. She also later headed up the Contracts Department for a time.

Denise remembers it was on a Sunday night that she received word that the operation was being sold to Biomedical Reference Laboratories in North Carolina.

The next day new faces appeared.

"I still remember the day they walked in the door. Jim [Powell] came in" with his management staff.

The first question was, "Who is in charge? ... What were the changes to be?"

At the time Denise said, "We were 'the lab' in our part of the country" and were facing an entirely different culture with the North Carolina company. "We were being paid a per diem of twenty-five dollars per day. It was seven dollars at BRL. There were big differences in northern and southern cultures," she said.

McFadden became the point person for her side of the merger for a couple of years before moving into the area dealing with contracts. When the PCR lab opened in 1990 in the Research Triangle in North Carolina, Denise went there as one of five sales representatives.

Soon after Tom Mac Mahon became president and CEO of LabCorp, the leadership began work on a strategic plan to take the company into the future. "Each division had to report and justify its existence" to the leadership team, McFadden said. "I worked in clinical trials, and my boss was fired the day before the presentations, and I was told" to make the presentation the next day. She remembers that she and colleague Danny Shoemaker worked into the night to get ready, and the next day she told the group "this [clinical trials] is a business LabCorp wants to be in."

And LabCorp stayed in that business and "gave us all we needed to grow." She sold HIV testing to pharmaceutical companies for about five years and left after some differences about the direction things were moving.

Then, after her year of travels, she joined Covance and ultimately returned to LabCorp.

When the LabCorp-Covance union came, McFadden was in a unique spot, having been on both sides of the fence, and she had some observations about that move.

"David King wanted to be in clinical trials in a bigger way, and he wanted to expand the diagnostic business into Europe," she said. "Covance was all over the world."

Later in 2015 LabCorp bought Safe Foods International Holdings along with its two operating companies, International Food Network and The National Food Laboratory. The companies joined Covance's Nutritional Chemistry and Food Safety Division.

The National Food Laboratory was a consulting and testing firm providing creative, practical, and science-based insights to solve food safety, quality, and product and process development challenges for the food industry, according to a news release at the time of the purchase.

The company continued its work with individual diseases in 2015, unveiling a new diabetes guide and making new studies into HIV-1 and hepatitis viruses.

LabCorp also announced a collaboration with Japan-based Sysmex Corp. to develop blood-based molecular aid to tumor diagnosis.

In a news release, Chairman and CEO King said, "Our expanded relationship with Sysmex furthers our ability to bring innovative technologies that assist in the development of new oncology treatments to patients and builds upon our core mission of improving health and improving lives."

In March 2016 Pathology Inc. became a part of LabCorp. The Torrance, California, medical testing and service company was a full-service independent women's health laboratory providing reproductive FDA donor testing as well as anatomic, molecular, and digital pathology services. The acquisition, which included Pathology's patient service centers used to conduct its medical testing and services business, showed that LabCorp was continuing to look to the future with an eye toward continued growth and broadening its lists of services to its customers.

In an article in the *Burlington Times-News,* King said, "The added capabilities of Pathology Inc. enhance our existing women's health offerings and support LabCorp's strategic vision to provide world-class diagnostics that improve health and improve lives."

King also said "The environment for complementary acquisitions is favorable, and we expect to continue to expand our geographic footprint, test menu, and unique capabilities in diagnostics, drug development, and food safety through disciplined acquisitions that generate attractive financial returns."

King himself was in the news in early 2016 when he was elected a trustee of Elon University. The Elon campus lies just west of LabCorp's York Court laboratories. The company has programs at the university, including the Elon Academy college access and success program for local high school students, and internships in Elon's nationally recognized Martha and Spencer Love School of Business.

Wes Elingburg has been a member of the Elon Board of Trustees since 2005. He was recently chairman of the board and was presented an honorary degree from the university in 2016.

Dr. Jim Powell is also a past chair of the board and recipient of an honorary degree. He is currently serving as a life member of the Elon board.

By April 2016 LabCorp was "the world's leading health-care diagnostics company," according to a report in the Burlington Times-News. The company was "providing comprehensive clinical laboratory services through LabCorp Diagnostics, and end-to-end drug development support through Covance Drug Development." The company recorded net revenue in excess of $8.5 billion in 2015, according to that report. CEO King said, "We are off to a terrific start" for 2016. He continued,

> Broad-based demand for the services of LabCorp Diagnostics and Covance Drug Development is evidence of our customers' enthusiasm for our different offerings. We continue to carry out our mission to improve health and improve lives through focus on three key strategic objectives—delivering world-class diagnostics, bringing innovative medicines to patients faster, and changing the way care is provided.

In an interview in 2016, King looked back at his near-decade tenure as CEO and president, citing two particular moves by the company as the most important events of those years.

First, he said, was the contract in 2007 with UnitedHealthCare. "That gave us a presence all across the nation." In that move, LabCorp became the exclusive nationwide laboratory for United Health Care, a ten-year contract that was a historic move for LabCorp. Second, he said that the Covance purchase in 2014–2015 had huge ramifications for LabCorp as it "made us global," a true international company.

Covance plays a major role in the development of new drugs, King said, as he explained a bit of that process. He said the first step is to test in animals, and then tests are made to determine basic toxicity to make sure it will not be fatal to a person.

Then the drug is tested in healthy human volunteers to determine any effects on the body, as in liver or kidney functions. If the drug is determined safe, then it moves into trials involving hundreds and maybe thousands of people around the world. If it is found safe and helps a person with disease, it is given approval. Covance, he said, covers the process from the very beginning up through commercialization of the drug.

LabCorp wanted Covance, he said, because it was a big laboratory system and "it would expand us globally in diagnostics and laboratory services."

King said, "We again had the courage to bet on ourselves. We transformed our company into the world's largest laboratory *and* the world's leading health-care diagnostics company."

On April 27, 2016, LabCorp's market cap was $12.9 billion with a share price of $127. Those figures had jumped from $8.699 billion and $102.58 only four months earlier on December 31, 2015.

When asked to discuss the toughest decisions he has had to make, King laughed and said, "Covance." He said that was a $6 billion decision, and "my career was on the line."

"Covance was hard to do," he said, citing that cost, "but it was the thing to do."

Actually, he said, the toughest thing he has faced was losing a contract with Aetna in 2007. That could have been handled in several ways, but he said, "We felt strongly if we burned bridges it would come back," so we helped them close out of the contract although it was difficult for LabCorp.

"What will LabCorp look like in twenty-five years?" King was asked.

"In twenty-five years we will have labs all over the world, and not just in drug development," as is the case now. The footprint in drug development and diagnostics will be bigger, he said, and just recently the company has moved into testing in the food industry, another area of future presence.

"We invest in new tools, new ideas, and stay ahead of the curve. We will not be different in appearance but will do more and do it in more locations."

There is a major problem on the horizon, he said. "The regulatory environment is becoming more aggressive" on matters of what the company can be paid for. The whole industry is being affected, he said, but "we do it right."

Looking further ahead, he said, "We are the biggest in the world, but our job in the next fifty years is to make sure we are still here."

King had high praise for his predecessors. He called them true visionaries.

"Jim Powell saw what laboratory testing could become," he said, "and Tom Mac Mahon saw what it could become if we capitalized on our scale and standardized our platform" in billing and other areas, focusing on cancer testing, and taking the company to new levels.

"They were years ahead of the rest of this industry," he said, noting that the company has had only three CEOs in its nearly fifty-year history.

In May 2016 the company announced a new test for colorectal cancer screening: the Epi pro-Colorectal test. The test was developed by Epigenomics AG in Germany and is available in the United States through an agreement with Polymedco. LabCorp became the first laboratory in the United States to offer this test.

Dr. Mark Brecher, chief medical officer for LabCorp Diagnostics, said this test is of major significance as it offers a new and more convenient and comfortable way of colon testing. In a news release he said, "Many people are not properly screened because they are reluctant to collect a stool sample or undergo a colonoscopy."

As a result, he said, thousands of people who need to be screened can use the Epi pro-Colorectal test in an effort to find possible colon cancer in its early stages when it can be more effectively treated.

LabCorp's lead director Robert E. Mittlestaedt Jr. said in a 2016 interview that the company has grown over the years because of many factors. As the industry consolidated, LabCorp was acquiring other companies, and it was paying attention to the growth of managed care and how it affected the industry. Also, he said, in the laboratories and services, "We built a great medical team to be sure we are in the lead."

In the days ahead, he said, "We have to integrate data and add value to doctors and patients" as the industry is changing rapidly and will continue to do so.

As lead director on a board of ten members, Mittlestaedt serves as a liaison between the board and CEO King. He reviews the agenda of meetings and performs other duties as required. He is Dean Emeritus of the School of Business at Arizona State University.

Pat Frele retired on May 6, 2016, as a vice president after having started in 1973 as a part-time temp who was trying to earn some money while looking for a teaching job.

Her first work was in Roche Clinical Labs in Raritan, New Jersey. She had graduated college with a degree in elementary education, but at that time it seemed there just were no teaching positions open in New Jersey.

At Roche, she was a clerk, she did time cards, and she handled petty cash accounts and verified deposits. After she worked a while, she was asked by management, "Do you want to stay?"

She said yes, she would stay, and she said, "I stayed ... and stayed ... and stayed, for forty-three years." By 1982 she had become manager of the billing department.

When Roche Clinical Labs joined Biomedical Reference Labs, it was obvious they needed a new billing system. Frele was on the committee to develop that system, and she became director over billing.

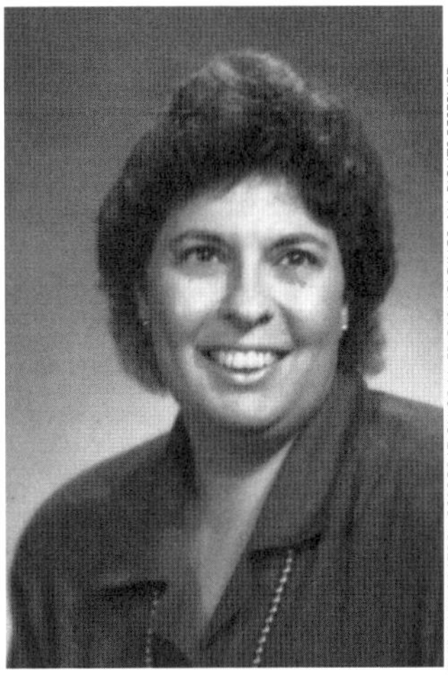

Pat Frele

Her duties had taken her to North Carolina, but in 1989–1990 the company created divisions of operations for the first time. She was asked if she wanted to move back to New Jersey into the Northeast Division. She did go back and was over finances for the division as well as customer services and the service center—in fact, over everything except sales and the laboratory department.

Frele had been a member of the conversion teams following the merger that created LabCorp, and she continued to have duties in that area until her retirement. She helped new companies that came into LabCorp through the conversion process to keep things running smoothly. In between her duties at work, she found time to earn her MBA degree. She moved back to Burlington in 2005, and as she retired, she said her career had been a great experience.

"If someone had told me I would go from being a clerk in that little company back in New Jersey to a vice president in a multi-billion dollar company today..." She did not finish the thought.

In 2016 Ben Miller had his hands full. He was executive vice president of the Atlantic Division, but he was also doing interim duty with the Mid-America and West Divisions and several other operations. Despite the extra duty, however, he was still enjoying his work after thirty-two years with the company.

He may have landed his first job in a more unique way than most any other employee. He literally chased down Jim Powell while Powell was stopped at a traffic signal in Greensboro. He had been calling to get an appointment with Powell but had not been successful.

He and a friend were on the street in Greensboro when his friend said, "That's Jim Powell," pointing to a car at the light. Miller took off at a run and tapped on the window.

It worked. Jim Powell set up an interview with Paul Hoffner and Linda Woody who was in human relations. Ben Miller went to work for the company on October 15, 1989.

He remembered that Jim Powell knew how to "pinch a penny." When traveling, employees doubled up in rooms with people they had never met before, "but it was okay," he said. "It created a frugal culture. We learned not to waste money."

Miller said there was a strong work ethic in the company: no-nonsense hard work, but "we were rewarded for it."

He said Jim Powell told him, "If you don't like change you won't like this business. That was very true. There had to be constant change to be successful, and we do it well. We embrace change."

Like many others, Miller used the word "visionary" in describing Jim Powell. Today, he said, throughout the industry there is a focus on helping doctors do a better job in treating their patients. Jim Powell was doing that in the 1980s. He was a real visionary."

In May 2016 the company announced another development described in a newspaper headline as a "cancer breakthrough."

The Food and Drug Administration had given approval to a new LabCorp test that would enhance the treatment for those suffering from bladder cancer.

The *Burlington Times-News* reported the approval of the Ventana PD-L1, a complementary diagnostic for Tecentriq, which immediately became available all across the nation. It is designed for immunotherapy treatment for patients with urothelial cancer, the most common malignancy of the urinary system and the ninth most common form of cancer in the world. Tecentriq is the first new therapy introduced for this type of cancer in the past thirty years, according to a news release from LabCorp. The test was developed by Roche Diagnostics.

LabCorp already has diagnostic tests to help identify patients who may benefit from new, targeted immunotherapy for the treatment of melanoma and lung cancer, according to the release.

Dr. Mark Brecher, LabCorp's chief medical officer, said the new assay "can help change the way care is provided by helping physicians better understand the potential benefits of treatment with Tecentriq for their patients with bladder cancer."

In that announcement, President and CEO David King said LabCorp is dedicated to improving health and improving lives through the introduction of new tests and by bringing innovative medicines to patients faster.

CHAPTER FIFTEEN

A True Life Sciences Company Emerges

THROUGHOUT ITS HISTORY, LabCorp has made steady progress toward becoming a life sciences company in the truest sense.

From LabCorp's very beginning, there have been dreams of morphing the organization into a new and unique company that would have special capabilities on the cutting edge of genetics testing. There was the desire to be part of scientific breakthroughs afforded by these capabilities. Today, the most promising prospect for LabCorp is to participate in the larger movement toward the development of customized, or novel, drugs and diagnostics for treatment of cancer and other diseases.

There are many strengths that put the company in this position, and it is interesting to see how they all fit together to bring LabCorp to its place as number one in the world. Some of these things have already been touched on in this book but deserve additional emphasis to properly place them in the historic progression toward that true biotechnology company.

LabCorp and its predecessors, going back to the Roche Biomedical Laboratories era, had a focus on growing the lab's capabilities in the area of DNA and genetics testing in general. RBL received a shot in the arm in 1991 when scientists at the parent company, F. Hoffmann–La Roche, recognized the potential in the work that had been done on DNA amplification at the Cetus Corporation in California.

Dr. Jurgen Drews, global research president for Roche, was one of the early proponents of PCR. Dr. Drews was in charge of human genomic studies at Roche for the development of novel drugs for cancer treatments and other maladies. When he and his team realized the true scope of what was going on at Cetus, Roche bought limited rights to the technology in 1989.

Kary Mullis, a future Nobel laureate who worked at Cetus with a group of scientists, had transformed the capability of the laboratory world by developing PCR to amplify DNA. This allowed for the actual testing of the DNA and the ability to quantitate this exquisite, minute substance found to be uniquely different in the cells of all humans, plants, and even prehistoric animals. Before PCR, DNA was present in such insufficient quantities that it could not be measured properly. Now, using PCR to actually amplify small quantities of DNA, a discarded cigarette at a crime scene could be linked to the suspect.

The greatest benefit from PCR, however, was to be useful in the discoveries and therapies for diagnosing and treating disease in humans.

One of the major steps that helped put LabCorp in its position in the industry today came when the parent company of Roche Biomedical Laboratories, under the guidance of Dr. Drews and his group, acquired worldwide rights to PCR from Cetus in 1991 for $300 million. Many less knowledgeable individuals could not imagine how Roche could spend such a sum for one type of lab-testing technology.

But when Roche spent that huge amount on PCR, the antennae of many scientists and their sponsors went up. The importance of PCR was then rapidly recognized, and there was immediate demand by the scientific community worldwide for access to this revolutionary technology.

An immediate debate began within Roche to properly determine how this technology should be managed. One small group advocated keeping access to PCR within the confines of the company and not releasing it to the general scientific community. With further discussion and feedback from prominent scientists outside the corporate walls, it was realized that this discovery was too big and too important for any one company to corner the market, nor would it want to.

Once the importance of this new ability to amplify DNA became more understood and widespread, competing techniques soon appeared, but none had the advantages of PCR—and the development of those technologies gradually disappeared in favor of PCR.

PCR: A Breakthrough for RBL

RBL was very much interested in PCR. The labs' scientists foresaw obvious and immediate applications, and this technology was to give the company the much sought-after head start in using PCR for the amplification of DNA.

That was when RBL immediately added the specialized PCR lab at its facility in Research Triangle Park in the Raleigh-Durham area of North Carolina. Dr. Myla Lai-Goldman headed the development of the new laboratory. This new PCR laboratory had to include a clean room with positive air pressure, much like one would find in a laminar flow hood. That precaution was necessary due to the risk of contamination of the PCR process in the early days of development. When completed, RBL had the premier facility in the world for performing PCR. The company immediately began using this unique technology to support the scientific community's interest in determining what could be accomplished by detecting and measuring DNA. Dr. Lai-Goldman spent many hours educating visitors to her laboratory.

The Research Triangle Park (RTP) facility had been established a few years earlier as the Center for Molecular Biology and Pathology to provide access to the extensive scientific community in that area. The original intentions of the company were to use this facility to build its capabilities in various specialty testing areas, particularly within genetics. Now it was adding the most critical component in that quest.

The first of the genetic testing laboratories at RTP had been for cytogenetics. The largest of the cytogenetics laboratories in the RBL network was moved south from Raritan, New Jersey, under the leadership of Dr. Raj Barathur. Cytogenetics testing was then consolidated under him. Dr. Barathur left the company later, and Dr. Tim Smith took a leadership role before Dr. Lai-Goldman arrived at the center.

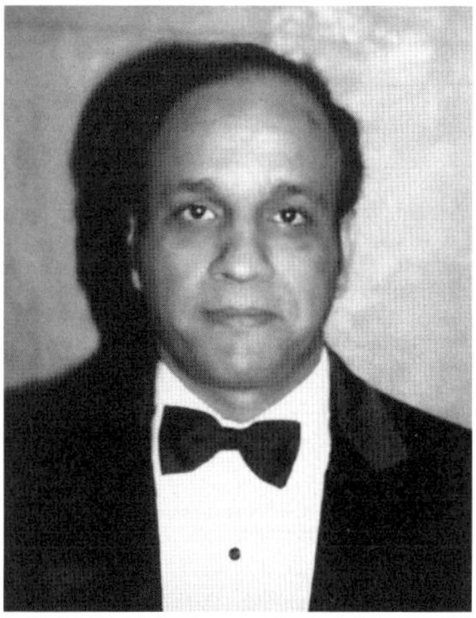

Dr. Raj Barathur

With the Roche acquisition of PCR, this RTP facility became the central testing point and training ground within the entire company. All testing using PCR was originally centralized at RTP, because of early requirements for the clean room and equipment and the knowledge base that was there for this complex procedure. As time passed, improvements in equipment were made that reduced the risk of contamination. The company then began setting up PCR testing facilities in other specialized laboratories within RBL to meet the increasing demand for tests utilizing PCR.

Paternity and Identification Testing

PCR technology led to new capabilities within RBL. The company already had a rather large division for forensic and paternity testing using certain laboratory technologies such as the human leukocyte antigen (HLA) testing, blood groups, and so on. These often nonconclusive procedures had led to extensive testimony by a group of scientists at RBL that specialized in court appearances to explain the arcane science available at that time. PCR changed all that as the scientific community and then the legal community began to understand and accept the power of DNA testing by PCR. As mentioned earlier, PCR allowed for the identification of US soldiers beginning with Operation Desert Storm so that remains of our military personnel no longer ended up in the Tomb of the Unknown Soldier in Washington, DC. There were no more unknowns.

Another application of PCR by LabCorp has been to identify the human papillomavirus (HPV) that causes cervical cancer as well as cancers of the lower gastrointestinal tract and the head and neck. For over forty years, cervical cancer had been detected by use of the Pap smear. It became the most successful cancer test in history and led to a great reduction in cervical cancer in the Western world. The Pap smear would soon be supplemented by detecting this causative agent for cervical cancer.

Researchers at the Rockefeller Institute (now Rockefeller University) in New York City, in working on the first oncogenic retrovirus, discovered in 1911 that viruses can cause cancer in chickens. Many years later it was discovered that HPV was the cause of cervical and other cancers in humans. The problem was that there was not a practical means of testing for HPV. PCR techniques solved this problem, and now hundreds of thousands of HPV cancer tests are performed at LabCorp each year to supplement the Pap smear.

PCR Helps Conquer AIDS

The conquest of the AIDS epidemic has been greatly aided by using PCR to detect the presence of the human immunodeficiency virus (HIV) that is responsible for the infection causing this disease. HIV was slow to be detected by the older, more traditional means of testing, such as looking for antibodies to the virus. New tests for HIV first developed at Cetus made it possible to diagnose AIDS at an extremely early stage, before the appearance of antibodies, so that treatment could begin earlier. Cetus also developed a method for detecting and monitoring the HIV viral load in an infected individual so that the effectiveness of a particular therapy could be monitored and adjusted if necessary. Due to these cutting-edge laboratory technologies and the development of drug cocktails and combinations, AIDS has now become a chronic disease that can be managed and treated; it is no longer a death sentence.

Prenatal testing has been revolutionized by new PCR-based technologies that are rapidly replacing amniocentesis in pregnant women, which is most often performed in those over thirty-five years of age. The primary focus has been to detect the trisomy-21 defect that leads to various levels of Down syndrome in affected newborns.

For many years, cells have been obtained by inserting a needle into the amniotic sac of a pregnant woman to withdraw a sample of fetal cells. This sample is then sent to the chromosome analysis laboratory for the actual culturing of the fetal cells. This is followed by the disrupting of the cell walls to harvest the chromosomes. These chromosomes are photographed; the images are cut out of the photo like paper dolls, arranged numerically, photographed again, and this image is interpreted by a cytogenetics expert. The procedure is known as karyotyping.

The new technology is to detect the fetal DNA that has crossed the placental barrier into the mother's circulation. The ability has been developed to test for, then statistically separate, maternal from fetal DNA and to look for genetic abnormalities that can be attributed to the fetus.

In 2016 LabCorp acquired Sequenom, which developed the first commercially available test of this type called a sequencing-based noninvasive chromosomal aneuploidy test. The second company to develop a similar test was Verinata, now owned by Illumina. Dr. Jim Powell helped found the predecessor company, Living Microsystems (LMS), that became Verinata. Sequemon and Illumina share intellectual property in a pooling arrangement and are the leading companies in this field.

Sequenom, as well as a number of other biotechnology companies, also has a liquid-based cancer detection test under development. The potential for this test remains to be seen, but it is an example of the increasing applications for cancer detection and differentiation made possible by DNa testing by PCR.

The Advent of Novel Drug Development

LabCorp has teamed with Hatteras Venture Partners to form a new company, Gene-Centric Diagnostics. LabCorp has made an investment and has a minority interest in the Company. This effort is directed by Drs. Chuck Perrou, Neil Hayes, and Dr. Myla Lai-Goldman. Dr. Lai-Goldman is the former medical officer and chief scientific officer at LabCorp and president of this new organization. The company is focused on enabling oncologists and their patients to make more informed, individualized treatment decisions. Providing molecular diagnostic testing is critical to knowing the genetic makeup and proper identification of a particular tumor. Tumors respond to treatment differently depending on their genetic constitution.

Other work in the laboratories of Drs. Perrou and Hayes at UNC–Chapel Hill has been on the classification of the diversity of breast tumors. This genomic-based classification is known as the "intrinsic subtypes of breast cancer." Dr. Perrou and his associates have shown that breast cancer can be subtyped into at least five molecular subtypes.

The Perrou work is cited as an example of how LabCorp's capabilities fit into the larger world of delivering novel and customized pharmaceuticals for cancer treatments. In the future, developments of these unique drugs and therapies will depend on laboratory testing in the beginning to determine the genetic and other characteristics of a tumor.

CHAPTER SIXTEEN

Plotting the Future of LabCorp

THE DEVELOPMENTS LISTED in the previous chapter are among the most important in the formation of the company that, in the second decade of the twenty-first century, has become the world leader in its field.

Now it is up to CEO Dave King, his management group, and the LabCorp Board of Directors to determine the company's strategic path as it moves into the future. The opportunities for LabCorp were and are multiple.

For instance, LabCorp has become one of the largest logistics companies in the world—certainly so within the health-care arena. Due to the nature of the commercial laboratory business as it has developed over the years, LabCorp has tens of thousands of direct contacts with health-care providers on a daily basis. Salespeople, specialists in specimen acquisition, and equipment maintenance and supplies specialists visit hospitals and physicians' offices to fulfill the complex needs of doctors, nurses, and other health-care providers. Thus there is tremendous value in a logistics company, especially as consolidation is accelerating in health care in the United States.

A Unique Information System in Health Care

There is huge value in the unique and widespread connectivity that LabCorp has within the world of information systems in health care. When a person goes to see a physician or to the hospital in this day and time, the proliferation of laptops and tablets is observed. These computers need to be connected to share information about a patient. This capability is certainly not reality yet, but in the future a specific doctor's office or hospital should be connected to all the other providers in a specific community, and with all other health-care providers who might need to see a specific patient.

LabCorp and its predecessors over the years have gone through the laborious, time-consuming, and expensive process of connecting its laboratories into one computer system with essentially all of the hospitals, clinics, and doctors' offices that it serves. This connectivity exists for tens of thousands of different providers. This process has been continuous over almost fifty years. The company began by reporting lab results via teletypes, then dumb computer terminals, and later smart terminals in the provider's location. More recently this communication has improved by having lab results go directly from the centralized computer at LabCorp to the patient's medical record at the provider location, wherever that might be.

Such connectivity on this scale is unique. The possibility for this centralized capability can be traced back to the business decisions made forty-seven years ago at Biomedical Laboratories in Burlington, North Carolina. The decision was to build a laboratory system that would always have a centralized computer system. This approach would be expensive and time consuming but would result in efficiency and better quality control.

As Biomedical Labs grew by expanding geographically, then by making acquisitions, new locations or acquired laboratories were always brought onto the centralized computer system. This computer consolidation was continued through the years of Roche Biomedical Laboratories. When NHL and RBL merged to form LabCorp, the extensive job of bringing their multiple and nonconsolidated laboratory networks onto the central legacy system from RBL was a massive undertaking, as Pat Frele mentioned.

As a result of this nearly fifty-year corporate-wide computer consolidation program, LabCorp has an extremely powerful tool to mine Big Data going forward. The future in health care is to be able to use Big Data for diagnostics, treatment, and drug development.

LabCorp had a large biorepository facility at the North Carolina Research Campus in Kannapolis, North Carolina, as well. There, hundreds of thousands of well-annotated specimens were stored, waiting to be part of the Big Data revolution. Operations there were closed in 2016 and consolidated with the Covance Biorepository in Greenfield, Indiana.

Quest Diagnostics

The only other independent laboratory that competes with LabCorp on a national scale continues to be Quest Diagnostics, begun the same year as LabCorp in 1969. Management at LabCorp has measured itself against Quest over many years, especially since both are on public exchanges with competitive information readily available.

There are other independent labs with equal or greater market share in various geographic markets, and various hospital laboratory systems, that compete on a very broad scale.

In recent times, financial analysts have compared the different routes on which the two companies have embarked. On the one hand, Quest is continuing to build its business as a commercial clinical laboratory expanding by more acquisitions in the same space of clinical laboratory testing. They have also ventured into acquiring clinical laboratories that have been run by the larger provider networks.

Analysts have contrasted the approach taken by Quest with that of LabCorp, especially since LabCorp's acquisition of Covance. Some of those analysts believe that Quest has set its course on becoming a larger commercial clinical laboratory with the possible risk of being viewed as a commodity. Some believe that companies that are considered commodities are ultimately of less value to society and to the investing public.

On the other hand, David King and his LabCorp team have obviously considered all the assets of LabCorp enumerated above. They have elected to take the route of creating a true life sciences company, building on the unique capabilities in the field of genetics developed over the years at LabCorp and its predecessors. This has been particularly aided by the early start that RBL and LabCorp had with PCR.

Fortunately, LabCorp has been highly profitable in recent years, generating large amounts of free cash. The financial community likes to see a highly profitable company use this to make acquisitions and to develop new and improved products and services that enhance the company's value.

This is what Dave King and his team did, striking the right note with a bold initiative into biotechnology with the Covance purchase, a move that will further enhance LabCorp's position as number one in the world in its industry.

Eyes to the Future

As LabCorp closes in on its fiftieth year, a company publication has reviewed the corporate mission as eyes are turned to the future:

> LabCorp provides leading-edge medical laboratory tests and services through a national network of primary clinical laboratories and specialty laboratories.
>
> LabCorp processes tests on approximately 470,000 specimens each day, applying advances in medicine and science to laboratory testing.
>
> LabCorp operates a sophisticated laboratory network, with corporate headquarters in Burlington, NC, and more than 50,000 employees worldwide. Our 220,000 clients include physician offices, hospitals, managed care organizations, and biotechnology and pharmaceutical companies.

Another company release stated, "At LabCorp, our commitment to scientific leadership ensures that clients have access to industry-leading expertise and the latest developments in medical diagnostics.

"With a test menu of more than 3,000 individual assays and a staff of more than 200 PhDs and MDs, LabCorp is a comprehensive reference source from esoteric testing to anatomic pathology. At the core of LabCorp's approach is its world-renowned Specialty Testing Group. Each specialty lab operates as the discipline hub for performing and developing specialized testing as well as establishing best practices throughout the LabCorp network."

Those specialty tests include genetics, oncology, coagulation, endocrinology, infectious diseases, and allergy-immunology.

Laboratory Corporation of America Holdings is listed on the New York Stock Exchange under ticker symbol LH.

Many of those who appear throughout this story marvel at the way the company evolved from three rooms in an old hospital to its current place as industry and world leader. Many who were part of that journey said, "It was a great ride."

But Robert E. Mittlestaedt Jr., lead director in 2016, might have summed it up best.

He referred back to the fact that all this started in a small town called Burlington in North Carolina, and now it has grown to cover the United States and many countries around the world. And then he said, "We are a long way from where we started."

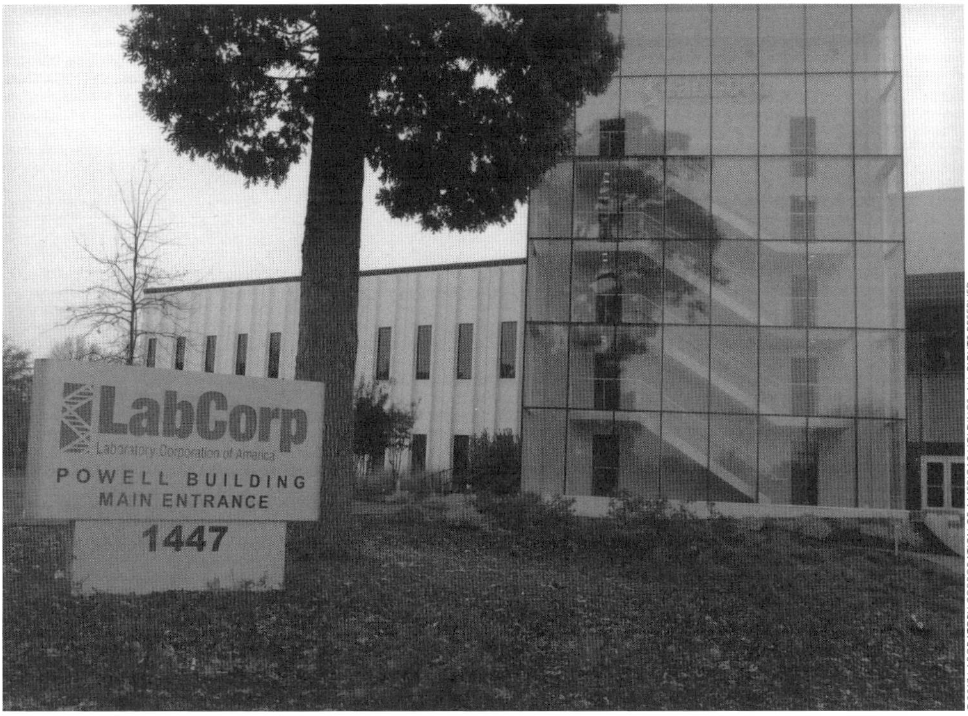

The modern Powell Building at York Court

ABOUT THE AUTHOR

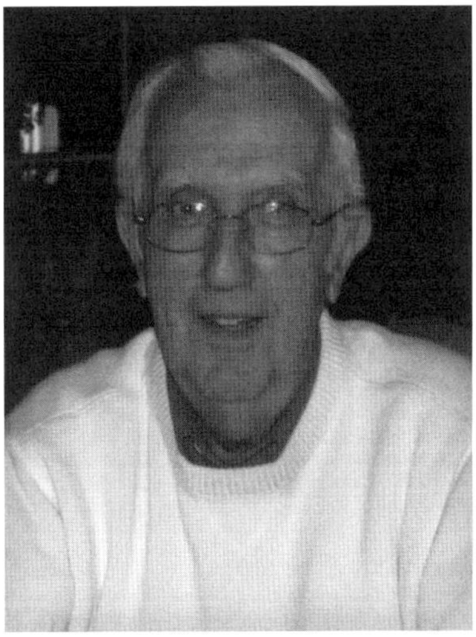

Don Bolden

Don Bolden is editor emeritus of the *Burlington (NC) Times-News,* where he spent fifty-one years, eighteen of them as executive editor. His newspaper career carried him to such interesting places as the Oval Office in the White House when President Reagan was in office and to the Soviet Union just days before the Berlin Wall started coming down. He is a Burlington native and a graduate of the University of North Carolina School of Journalism. He has produced twelve previous books, all related to Alamance County history. His wife of sixty years, the former Billie Faye Johnson, died in 2017. Don continues to reside in Burlington, his hometown.

Dr. Jim Powell lives in retirement in Burlington just a short distance from the York Court Laboratory. He is married to the former Anne Ellington and they have three children, John Banks Powell, James Rosser Powell and Helen Bobbitt Powell. He also has a daughter, Daphne Powell Markcrow, from his marriage to Pamela Oughton.